Weight Watchers

New Complete Cookbook

Simple and Satisfying Updated WW Recipes with Points Values
to Help You Achieve Your Weight Loss Goals Effortlessly |
Including a 30-day Meal Plan (FULL COLOR IMAGES)

Kathryn brandl

Disclaimer:

The information in this book is intended for informational purposes only. The author and publisher make no representations or warranties with respect to the accuracy or completeness of the contents of this book, and the author and publisher shall not be liable for any damages arising from the use of the information contained herein. Readers are encouraged to use their own judgment and consult with a professional if needed, especially in matters of health, nutrition, or diet.

Scan the QR code below to unlock your 5 bonuses!

Content

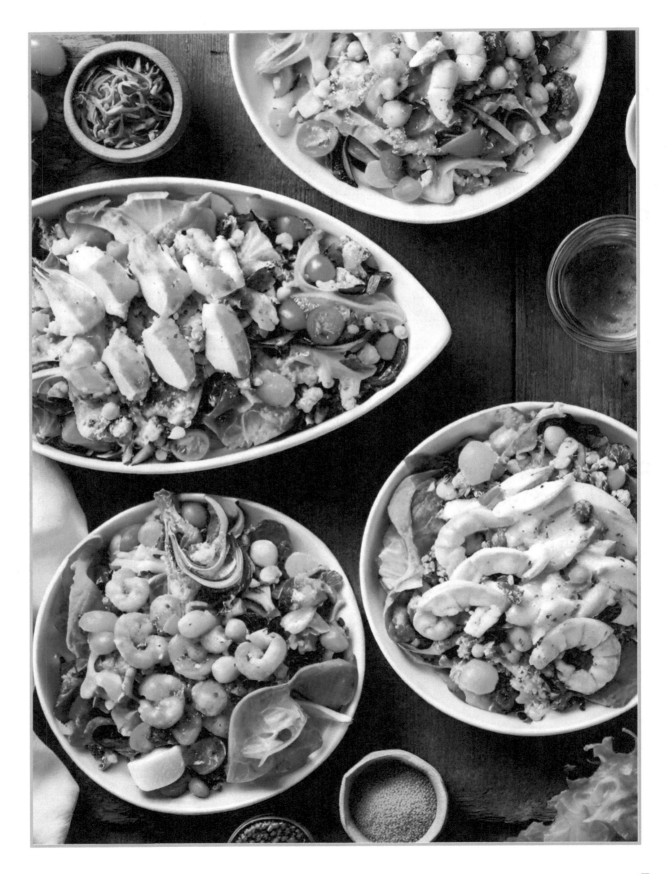

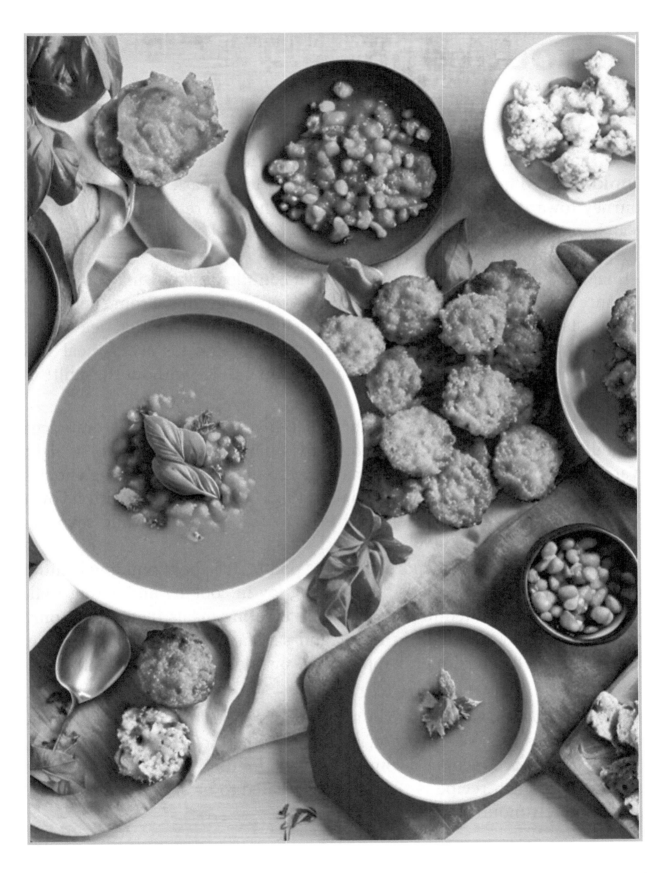

Introduction

Welcome to Weight Watchers

Hey there, and welcome to **"Weight Watchers New Complete Cookbook!"** I'm so excited you've decided to embark on this delicious journey toward your weight loss goals. Whether you're a seasoned Weight Watchers member or just starting out, this cookbook is designed to be your trusty companion every step of the way.

—Imagine stepping into your kitchen with confidence, knowing you have a treasure trove of tasty, satisfying recipes at your fingertips. From energizing breakfasts that kickstart your day to delightful dinners that leave you feeling nourished and content, we've got something for every meal and every mood. And yes, even desserts that let you indulge without the guilt!

Why Weight Watchers?

Weight Watchers isn't just another diet—it's a lifestyle that embraces flexibility, balance, and most importantly, enjoyment. The core of Weight Watchers is its Points system, a smart way to make mindful eating choices without feeling restricted. Each recipe in this cookbook comes with its own Points value, making it easier than ever to stay on track while savoring every bite.

—But Weight Watchers is more than just points. It's about building healthy habits, discovering new foods, and finding joy in cooking and eating well. This cookbook is crafted to support you in creating meals that are not only low in points but also high in flavor and satisfaction. Think of it as your personal guide to a healthier, happier you—one delicious recipe at a time.

What You'll Find Inside

Inside these pages, you'll discover a variety of recipes that cater to different tastes and lifestyles. Whether you're craving something sweet for breakfast, a hearty salad for lunch, or a comforting soup for dinner, there's something here for you. Each recipe is thoughtfully created to be simple, wholesome, and absolutely mouthwatering.

But that's not all! To make your journey even smoother, we've included a 30-day meal plan. This plan is your roadmap to success, offering a balanced mix of meals that keep you energized and satisfied throughout the month. Plus, with full-color images to inspire your culinary creations, you'll feel like a gourmet chef in your own kitchen.

Let's Get Started

Ready to dive in? Grab your apron, gather your ingredients, and let's make some magic happen in the kitchen. Whether you're cooking for yourself, your family, or friends, these recipes are here to make healthy eating easy and enjoyable. Remember, every great journey begins with a single step (or in this case, a single delicious bite).

—'Together, we'll explore new flavors, discover favorite go-to dishes, and celebrate every milestone along the way. Here's to a flavorful adventure and the wonderful results that await you. Let's make your weight loss goals not just achievable, but truly delightful!

Understanding Points

Navigating the Weight Watchers journey begins with a fundamental understanding of the Points system, a cornerstone of the program designed to simplify healthy eating without the stress of meticulous calorie counting. The Points system assigns a value to every food and beverage based on its nutritional content, including calories, protein, sugar, and saturated fat. This approach encourages mindful eating, allowing you to make informed choices that align with your weight loss goals.

—At its core, the Points system is about balance and flexibility. Instead of labeling foods as strictly "good" or "bad," it recognizes that all foods can fit into a healthy diet when consumed in appropriate portions. This means you can enjoy a wide variety of foods, from nutrient-dense vegetables to occasional indulgent treats, all while staying within your personalized daily Points budget.

Your daily Points allowance is tailored to your individual profile, taking into account factors such as age, gender, weight, height, and activity level. This personalized budget ensures that your weight loss plan is sustainable and effective, providing the right amount of flexibility to suit your lifestyle. By tracking your Points, you gain the freedom to choose meals that you love without feeling restricted or deprived.

—One of the standout features of the Points system is the inclusion of ZeroPoint foods. These are nutritious, low-calorie options that you can enjoy without tracking or counting towards your daily Points total. Foods like fresh fruits, vegetables, lean proteins, and whole grains fall into this category, allowing you to fill your plate with wholesome ingredients that keep you satisfied and energized throughout the day. Incorporating ZeroPoint foods into your meals is a strategic way to maximize your Points budget, ensuring you stay full and nourished while making room for other delicious choices.

Tracking your Points is straightforward, especially with the recipes in this cookbook clearly labeled with their respective Points values. This transparency simplifies meal planning, enabling you to effortlessly incorporate these dishes into your daily routine. Each recipe is crafted to be both flavorful and mindful of your Points, ensuring that you can enjoy every bite without the hassle of complex calculations.

To make the most of the Points system, consider these strategies:

1. **Start with ZeroPoint Foods**: Begin your meals with a generous serving of vegetables or a fresh salad. This not only helps you feel full but also allows you to use your Points for more substantial or indulgent items later in the meal.

2. **Mind Your Portions**: Even when enjoying higher-Point foods, being mindful of portion sizes can help you stay within your daily budget. Using measuring tools or portion control plates can be beneficial in maintaining balance.

3. **Plan Ahead**: Utilize the 30-day meal plan included in this cookbook to organize your meals in advance. Planning helps ensure a balanced distribution of Points throughout the day and week, reducing the likelihood of impulsive, higher-Point food choices.

4. **Stay Hydrated**: Drinking plenty of water is essential for overall health and can help manage hunger levels. Sometimes, what feels like hunger is actually thirst, so keeping hydrated can prevent unnecessary Points consumption.

5. **Enjoy Treats Wisely**: It's perfectly okay to indulge occasionally. When you do, savor each bite and enjoy the experience without guilt. Being mindful about treats ensures they remain a joyful part of your diet rather than a source of stress.

The beauty of the Points system lies in its adaptability. Whether you're preparing a quick weekday meal or planning a special weekend dinner, the system accommodates your needs, allowing you to enjoy a diverse range of foods while progressing toward your weight loss goals. This flexibility fosters a positive relationship with food, transforming eating into an enjoyable and sustainable part of your lifestyle.

Meal Planning Tips

Embarking on your Weight Watchers journey is exciting, and effective meal planning can make all the difference in achieving your goals smoothly and enjoyably. Let me share some practical and inspiring tips to help you organize your meals, save time, and stay on track without feeling overwhelmed.

Start with a Weekly Overview

Begin by setting aside a little time each week to map out your meals. Think of it as creating a roadmap for your week ahead. Jot down what you'll have for breakfast, lunch, dinner, and snacks each day. This simple step can reduce the stress of deciding what to eat every morning and help you make mindful choices that align with your Points budget.

Embrace Variety

Variety is the spice of life, and it's especially important in meal planning. Incorporate a mix of proteins, vegetables, grains, and healthy fats into your meals to keep things interesting and nutritionally balanced. Try exploring different cuisines and cooking techniques to discover new favorite dishes.

This not only keeps your meals exciting but also ensures you're getting a wide range of nutrients.

Batch Cooking and Prep

One of the biggest time-savers in meal planning is batch cooking. Choose a day or a few hours each week to prepare ingredients in bulk. Cook grains like quinoa or brown rice, roast a variety of vegetables, and prepare proteins such as chicken breasts or tofu. Store these in airtight containers in the fridge, and you'll have the building blocks for quick and easy meals throughout the week. This method minimizes daily cooking time and makes it easier to assemble healthy meals even on your busiest days.

Smart Grocery Shopping

A well-thought-out grocery list is your best friend when it comes to meal planning. Before heading to the store, review your weekly meal plan and create a detailed shopping list organized by sections of the store. This not only ensures you have everything you need but also helps you avoid impulse buys that can derail your Points budget. Stick to your list as much as possible, and consider shopping the perimeter of the store where fresh produce, lean proteins, and whole grains are typically located.

Balance Your Plate

Each meal should be a harmonious balance of proteins, carbohydrates, and healthy fats to keep you satisfied and energized. Start by filling half your plate with non-starchy vegetables, a quarter with lean protein, and the remaining quarter with whole grains or starchy vegetables. This visual guide can help you create balanced meals effortlessly, ensuring you get the nutrients you need without overloading on any one component.

Plan for Leftovers

Cooking larger portions and planning for leftovers is a smart way to save both time and Points. Prepare double batches of dinners like soups, stews, or casseroles, and enjoy them as lunches the next day. Leftovers are not only convenient but also reduce food waste and make it easier to stick to your meal plan without the temptation of ordering takeout or grabbing something less healthy on the go.

Incorporate Flexibility

Life is unpredictable, and your meal plan should be flexible enough to accommodate changes. Allow yourself some wiggle room by including a few free-choice meals or having backup options ready. If something unexpected comes up, you can easily swap a meal without feeling stressed or derailed. The key is to stay adaptable and not view your meal plan as a rigid structure but rather as a supportive framework that guides you toward your goals.

Utilize the 30-Day Meal Plan

To give you a head start, this cookbook includes a thoughtfully designed 30-day meal plan. This plan offers a variety of meals that cater to different tastes and preferences, ensuring you never get bored. Each day is carefully balanced to provide the right mix of nutrients and Points, making it easier for you to stay on track without feeling restricted. Follow the meal plan as a guideline, and feel free to tweak it according to your personal preferences and schedule.

Keep It Simple

Simplicity is key to sustainable meal planning. Opt for recipes with minimal ingredients and straightforward instructions, especially when you're short on time. Simple meals can be just as delicious and satisfying as more complex dishes, and they make the cooking process enjoyable rather than daunting. Remember, the goal is to create a meal plan that fits seamlessly into your life, not to add extra stress.

Stay Inspired

Keeping your meal plan exciting and enjoyable is crucial for long-term success. Regularly seek inspiration from the diverse range of recipes in this cookbook. Try something new each week, experiment with different spices and herbs, and don't be afraid to put your own twist on a dish. When you look forward to your meals, sticking to your plan becomes much easier and more enjoyable.

Monitor and Adjust

As you progress on your Weight Watchers journey, take time to review how your meal planning is working for you. Are there certain meals you love more than others? Do you find yourself needing more variety or simplicity? Adjust your meal plan accordingly to better suit your evolving tastes and lifestyle. This ongoing process ensures that your meal planning remains effective and enjoyable, keeping you motivated and aligned with your weight loss goals.

Stay Organized

Use tools that help you stay organized, such as meal planning apps, calendars, or even a simple notebook. Keeping track of your meals, shopping lists, and prep schedules can help you stay on top of your plan and avoid last-minute stress. Find a system that works best for you and stick with it, making meal planning a seamless part of your routine.

Enjoy the Process

Lastly, remember to enjoy the process of meal planning and cooking. View it as an opportunity to nourish your body, explore new flavors, and express your creativity in the kitchen. When you approach meal planning with a positive mindset, it becomes a rewarding and fulfilling part of your weight loss journey.

Chapter 1: Breakfasts

Starting your day with a nutritious and satisfying breakfast sets the tone for the rest of your meals. These Weight Watchers-friendly recipes are designed to be both delicious and easy to prepare, ensuring you have the energy and motivation to tackle your day ahead. Whether you prefer something sweet or savory, these breakfasts will keep you aligned with your weight loss goals while delighting your taste buds.

Berry Almond Oats

There's nothing quite like a warm bowl of oatmeal to start your morning, and this Berry Almond Oats recipe takes it to the next level. Packed with fresh berries and the delightful crunch of almonds, it's a perfect blend of sweetness and texture that will keep you satisfied until lunch.

- Prep Time: 5 minutes
- Cook Time: 10 minutes
- Total Time: 15 minutes
- Servings: 2

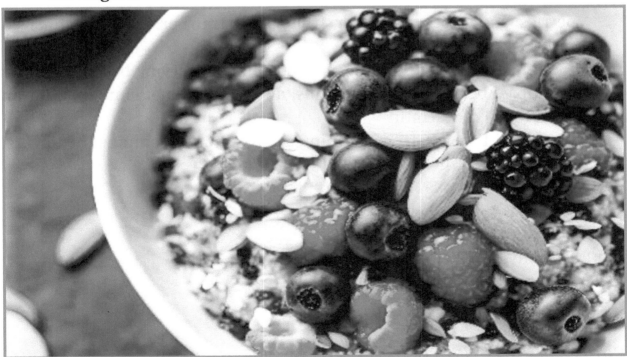

Ingredients:

- 1 cup old-fashioned rolled oats
- 2 cups unsweetened almond milk
- 1 tablespoon chia seeds
- 1 teaspoon vanilla extract
- 1 tablespoon honey or maple syrup (optional)
- 1 cup mixed fresh berries (such as strawberries, blueberries, raspberries)
- 2 tablespoons sliced almonds
- A pinch of cinnamon

Instructions:

1. Cook the Oats: In a medium saucepan, combine the rolled oats and almond milk. Bring to a gentle boil over medium heat, stirring occasionally.
2. Add Flavors: Once the mixture starts to simmer, stir in the chia seeds, vanilla extract, and honey or maple syrup if you're using it. Reduce the heat to low and let it cook for about 5 minutes, or until the oats are creamy and have absorbed most of the milk.
3. Prepare the Toppings: While the oats are cooking, rinse your fresh berries and slice any larger fruits like strawberries into bite-sized pieces.
4. Assemble the Bowl: Pour the cooked oats into serving bowls. Top with the mixed berries, sliced almonds, and a sprinkle of cinnamon for an extra touch of warmth.
5. Serve and Enjoy: Give everything a gentle mix to combine the flavors, and enjoy your hearty and delicious breakfast!

Nutrition Information (per serving):

- Calories: 250
- Protein: 7g
- Carbohydrates: 40g
- Fat: 8g
- Fiber: 8g
- Sugar: 12g

Points Value: 7 WW Points per serving

Tips & Variations:

- Nut-Free Option: Replace almonds with pumpkin seeds or sunflower seeds for a nut-free version.
- Sweetness Level: Adjust the amount of honey or maple syrup based on your sweetness preference or omit it altogether for a lower Points option.
- Extra Protein: Stir in a scoop of your favorite protein powder to boost the protein content and keep you fuller longer.

Start your day strong with this vibrant and nourishing bowl of Berry Almond Oats. The combination of fiber-rich oats and antioxidant-packed berries not only satisfies your taste buds but also fuels your body with essential nutrients. Enjoy this delightful breakfast knowing you're making a positive choice for your health and weight loss journey.

Spinach Feta Muffins

Kickstart your day with these savory Spinach Feta Muffins. They're perfect for those who prefer a hearty, protein-packed breakfast that's both tasty and convenient. Plus, they're easy to make ahead, making your mornings a breeze.

- Prep Time: 15 minutes
- Cook Time: 25 minutes
- Total Time: 40 minutes
- Servings: 12 muffins

Ingredients:

- 2 cups whole wheat flour
- 1 tablespoon baking powder
- 1/2 teaspoon salt
- 1/2 teaspoon black pepper
- 1 teaspoon dried oregano
- 1 cup fresh spinach, finely chopped

- 1/2 cup crumbled feta cheese
- 1/4 cup grated Parmesan cheese
- 1 cup low-fat Greek yogurt
- 2 large eggs
- 1/4 cup milk (dairy or non-dairy)
- 2 tablespoons olive oil

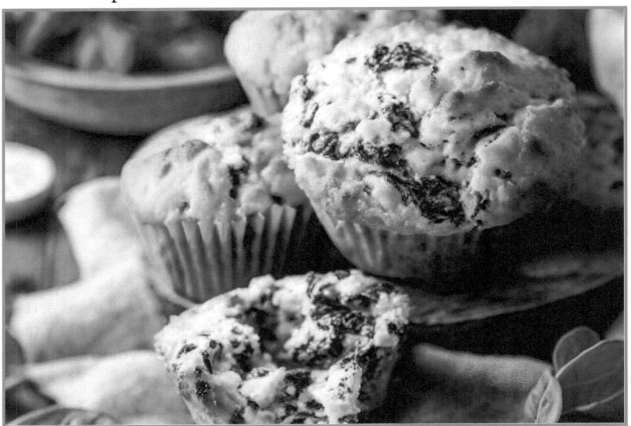

Instructions:

1. Preheat the Oven: Preheat your oven to 375°F (190°C). Line a muffin tin with paper liners or lightly grease it with cooking spray.
2. Mix Dry Ingredients: In a large bowl, whisk together the whole wheat flour, baking powder, salt, black pepper, and dried oregano.
3. Add Vegetables and Cheese: Fold in the finely chopped spinach, crumbled feta cheese, and grated Parmesan cheese until they are evenly distributed throughout the dry mixture.
4. Combine Wet Ingredients: In another bowl, whisk together the Greek yogurt, eggs, milk, and olive oil until smooth and well combined.

5. Combine Wet and Dry Mixtures: Pour the wet ingredients into the dry ingredients and stir until just combined. Be careful not to overmix; a few lumps are okay.
6. Fill the Muffin Tin: Divide the batter evenly among the prepared muffin cups, filling each about three-quarters full.
7. Bake to Perfection: Place the muffin tin in the preheated oven and bake for 20-25 minutes, or until the tops are golden brown and a toothpick inserted into the center comes out clean.
8. Cool and Serve: Allow the muffins to cool in the tin for a few minutes before transferring them to a wire rack to cool completely. Enjoy warm or store them in an airtight container for up to five days.

Nutrition Information (per muffin):

- Calories: 110
- Protein: 5g
- Carbohydrates: 12g
- Fat: 5g
- Fiber: 2g
- Sugar: 1g

Points Value: 3 WW Points per muffin

Tips & Variations:

- Make Ahead: These muffins freeze well. Simply wrap them individually and store in the freezer for a quick grab-and-go breakfast.
- Add Veggies: Feel free to add other vegetables like diced bell peppers or shredded zucchini for extra nutrition and flavor.
- Cheese Alternatives: Swap feta for goat cheese or a reduced-fat cheddar to change up the flavor profile or reduce the Points value.

These Spinach Feta Muffins are a savory delight that not only taste amazing but also provide a solid protein boost to keep you energized throughout the morning. Their versatility makes them a perfect make-ahead option, ensuring you have a wholesome breakfast ready even on your busiest days.

Protein Smoothie Bowls

Kickstart your morning with a vibrant and nutrient-packed Protein Smoothie Bowl. This recipe blends the creaminess of Greek yogurt with the freshness of fruits and the satisfying texture of granola, providing a balanced and energizing start to your day.

- Prep Time: 10 minutes
- Cook Time: 0 minutes
- Total Time: 10 minutes
- Servings: 2

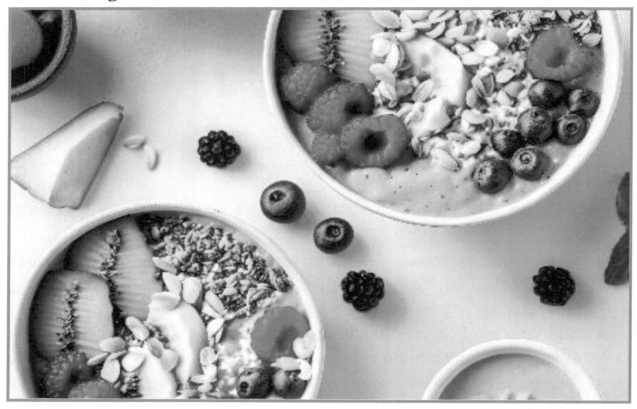

Ingredients:

- 1 cup unsweetened almond milk
- 1 cup low-fat Greek yogurt
- 1 banana, frozen
- 1/2 cup frozen mixed berries (such as strawberries, blueberries, and raspberries)
- 1 tablespoon almond butter

- 1 scoop vanilla protein powder
- 1 tablespoon chia seeds
- 1/2 teaspoon vanilla extract
- Toppings:
- 1/4 cup granola (low-sugar variety)
- 1/4 cup fresh berries
- 1 tablespoon sliced almonds
- A drizzle of honey or maple syrup (optional)

Instructions:

1. Blend the Base: In a blender, combine the unsweetened almond milk, low-fat Greek yogurt, frozen banana, frozen mixed berries, almond butter, vanilla protein powder, chia seeds, and vanilla extract. Blend until smooth and creamy. If the mixture is too thick, add a little more almond milk to reach your desired consistency.
2. Pour and Smooth: Pour the smoothie mixture into two serving bowls, creating a smooth and even surface.
3. Add Toppings: Top each bowl with granola, fresh berries, sliced almonds, and a light drizzle of honey or maple syrup if desired. These toppings add a delightful crunch and extra flavor to your smoothie bowl.
4. Serve Immediately: Enjoy your Protein Smoothie Bowl immediately for the best texture and freshness.

Nutrition Information (per serving):

- Calories: 300
- Protein: 20g
- Carbohydrates: 35g
- Fat: 10g
- Fiber: 7g
- Sugar: 18g

Points Value: 8 WW Points per serving

Tips & Variations:

- Dairy-Free Option: Substitute Greek yogurt with a plant-based yogurt to make this recipe dairy-free.

- Flavor Boost: Add a handful of spinach or kale for an extra boost of greens without altering the taste significantly.
- Different Protein: Use your favorite flavor of protein powder, such as chocolate or berry, to change up the flavor profile.
- Low-Sugar Toppings: Opt for unsweetened granola or reduce the amount of honey/maple syrup to lower the Points value.

This Protein Smoothie Bowl is not only visually appealing with its vibrant colors but also packed with essential nutrients to keep you full and focused throughout the morning. The combination of protein, fiber, and healthy fats ensures a balanced meal that supports your weight loss journey while satisfying your taste buds.

Avocado Toast

Simple yet incredibly satisfying, Avocado Toast is a timeless breakfast favorite that combines creamy avocado with hearty whole grain bread. This version adds a flavorful twist with cherry tomatoes and a sprinkle of feta cheese, making it both delicious and Weight Watchers-friendly.

- Prep Time: 5 minutes
- Cook Time: 5 minutes
- Total Time: 10 minutes
- Servings: 2

Ingredients:

- 4 slices whole grain or sprouted bread
- 1 ripe avocado
- 1/2 cup cherry tomatoes, halved
- 2 tablespoons crumbled feta cheese
- 1 tablespoon lemon juice
- 1 clove garlic, minced (optional)
- Salt and pepper to taste
- Red pepper flakes or fresh herbs (such as basil or cilantro) for garnish

Instructions:

1. Toast the Bread: Begin by toasting the slices of whole grain or sprouted bread to your desired level of crispiness. This provides a sturdy base for the creamy avocado topping.

2. Prepare the Avocado: While the bread is toasting, cut the ripe avocado in half, remove the pit, and scoop the flesh into a bowl. Mash the avocado with a fork until it's smooth but still has a bit of texture.

3. Add Flavor: Stir in the lemon juice, minced garlic (if using), and a pinch of salt and pepper into the mashed avocado. This adds brightness and depth of flavor to the spread.

4. Assemble the Toast: Spread the seasoned avocado evenly onto each slice of toasted bread. Top with halved cherry tomatoes and sprinkle crumbled feta cheese over the top.

5. Garnish and Serve: Add a dash of red pepper flakes or your favorite fresh herbs for an extra burst of flavor and visual appeal. Serve immediately and enjoy!

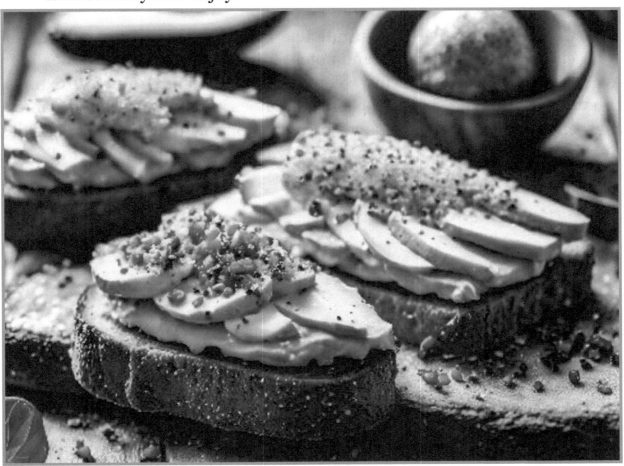

Nutrition Information (per serving):

- Calories: 220
- Protein: 6g
- Carbohydrates: 28g
- Fat: 12g
- Fiber: 7g
- Sugar: 4g

Points Value: 5 WW Points per serving

Tips & Variations:

- Add Protein: Top your avocado toast with a poached or boiled egg for an extra protein boost, increasing the Points value by 2-3.
- Spice It Up: Incorporate a drizzle of sriracha or hot sauce for a spicy kick without adding many Points.
- Veggie Boost: Add slices of cucumber or radish for added crunch and nutrition.
- Cheese Alternatives: Substitute feta with goat cheese or a reduced-fat cheese to vary the flavor and potentially reduce the Points value.

Avocado Toast is the perfect blend of creamy and crunchy textures, enhanced by the juicy burst of cherry tomatoes and the savory notes of feta cheese. It's a versatile and quick breakfast option that not only satisfies your hunger but also keeps you aligned with your Weight Watchers Points, making it a go-to choice for busy mornings.

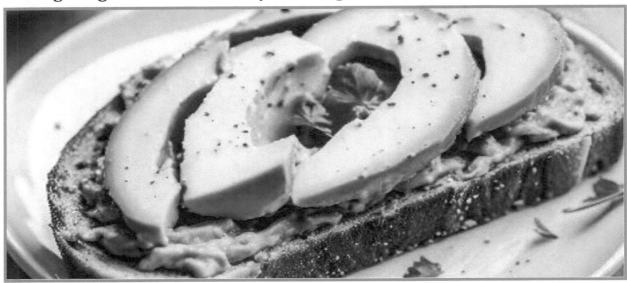

Chapter 2: Salads

Salads are no longer just a side dish—they can be the star of the meal when prepared thoughtfully. These Weight Watchers-friendly salad recipes combine fresh ingredients with bold flavors to create dishes that are light, nourishing, and incredibly satisfying. Whether you're looking for a hearty protein-packed option or a refreshing vegetarian delight, these salads are sure to please.

Chicken Caesar Salad

This lighter version of the classic Chicken Caesar Salad offers all the bold flavors you love, without the guilt. Crispy romaine, juicy grilled chicken, and a tangy homemade dressing come together for a salad that's perfect for lunch or dinner.

- Prep Time: 10 minutes
- Cook Time: 15 minutes
- Total Time: 25 minutes
- Servings: 2

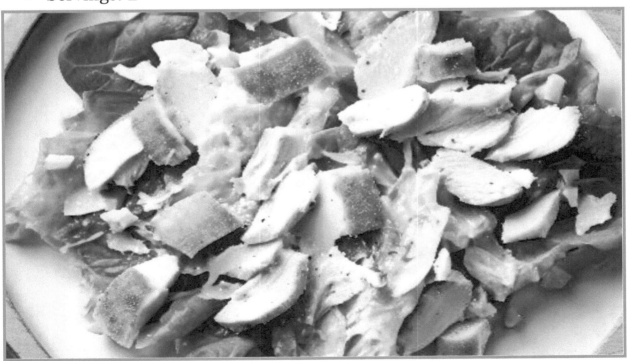

Ingredients:

- 2 boneless, skinless chicken breasts
- 1 teaspoon olive oil
- 1 teaspoon garlic powder
- Salt and pepper to taste
- 4 cups chopped romaine lettuce
- 1/2 cup cherry tomatoes, halved
- 1/4 cup grated Parmesan cheese
- 1/4 cup whole-grain croutons

Dressing:

- 2 tablespoons low-fat Greek yogurt
- 1 tablespoon Dijon mustard
- 1 teaspoon Worcestershire sauce
- 1 teaspoon lemon juice
- 1 clove garlic, minced
- Salt and pepper to taste

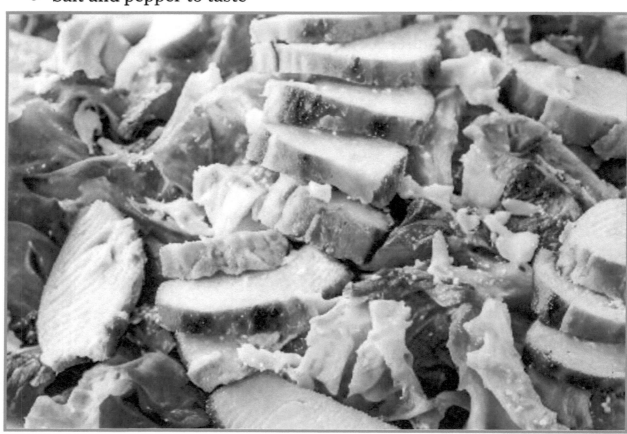

Instructions:

1. Prepare the Chicken: Rub the chicken breasts with olive oil, garlic powder, salt, and pepper. Grill or pan-sear them over medium heat for about 6-8 minutes per side, or until fully cooked. Allow the chicken to rest for 5 minutes before slicing.
2. Make the Dressing: In a small bowl, whisk together the Greek yogurt, Dijon mustard, Worcestershire sauce, lemon juice, minced garlic, salt, and pepper until smooth. Adjust the seasoning to taste.
3. Assemble the Salad: In a large bowl, toss the chopped romaine lettuce and cherry tomatoes with the dressing until evenly coated.
4. Add the Toppings: Divide the salad into two bowls. Top each with sliced grilled chicken, grated Parmesan cheese, and whole-grain croutons.
5. Serve and Enjoy: Serve immediately for the freshest flavors and textures.

Nutrition Information (per serving):

- Calories: 300
- Protein: 35g
- Carbohydrates: 15g
- Fat: 10g
- Fiber: 4g
- Sugar: 3g

Points Value: 7 WW Points per serving

Tips & Variations:

- Vegetarian Option: Replace the chicken with grilled tofu or chickpeas for a vegetarian version.
- Extra Veggies: Add sliced cucumbers or roasted red peppers for added crunch and flavor.
- Crouton Alternative: Swap croutons for toasted nuts or seeds to reduce carbohydrates and add healthy fats.

This Chicken Caesar Salad delivers all the satisfying flavors of the classic dish, with a healthy twist. Perfectly grilled chicken and a creamy dressing make it a go-to salad for any occasion. Enjoy every bite knowing it's both delicious and aligned with your weight loss goals.

Quinoa Veggie Salad

This vibrant Quinoa Veggie Salad is a nutritional powerhouse packed with protein, fiber, and fresh vegetables. It's a versatile dish that works as a light main course or a hearty side dish.

- Prep Time: 15 minutes
- Cook Time: 15 minutes
- Total Time: 30 minutes
- Servings: 4

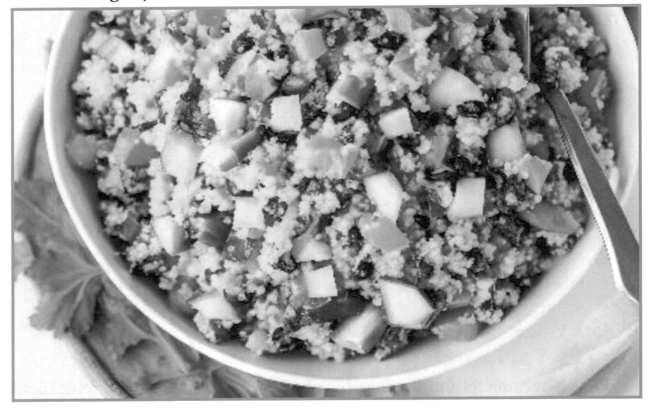

Ingredients:

- 1 cup quinoa
- 2 cups water or low-sodium vegetable broth
- 1 cup cherry tomatoes, halved
- 1 cup diced cucumber
- 1/2 cup shredded carrots
- 1/4 cup chopped red onion
- 1/4 cup fresh parsley, chopped

- 1/4 cup crumbled feta cheese
- 2 tablespoons olive oil
- 1 tablespoon lemon juice
- 1 teaspoon red wine vinegar
- Salt and pepper to taste

Instructions:

1. Cook the Quinoa: Rinse the quinoa under cold water to remove any bitterness. In a medium saucepan, bring the water or vegetable broth to a boil. Add the quinoa, reduce the heat to low, cover, and simmer for about 15 minutes or until the liquid is absorbed. Fluff with a fork and let cool.
2. Prepare the Vegetables: While the quinoa cools, chop the cherry tomatoes, cucumber, carrots, red onion, and parsley.
3. Make the Dressing: In a small bowl, whisk together the olive oil, lemon juice, red wine vinegar, salt, and pepper.
4. Combine Ingredients: In a large mixing bowl, combine the cooked quinoa, vegetables, and feta cheese. Pour the dressing over the top and toss until well combined.
5. Serve and Enjoy: Divide the salad into serving bowls and garnish with additional parsley or feta cheese if desired.

Nutrition Information (per serving):

- Calories: 240
- Protein: 8g
- Carbohydrates: 30g
- Fat: 10g
- Fiber: 5g
- Sugar: 3g

Points Value: 6 WW Points per serving

Tips & Variations:

- Add Protein: Incorporate grilled chicken, shrimp, or chickpeas for a more filling meal.
- Herb Swap: Substitute parsley with cilantro or dill for a different flavor profile.

- Meal Prep: This salad keeps well in the fridge for up to three days, making it a great option for meal prep.

This Quinoa Veggie Salad is as colorful as it is nutritious. Packed with fresh vegetables and hearty quinoa, it's a meal that will leave you feeling energized and satisfied. Enjoy it as a light lunch or a vibrant side dish that's sure to impress.

Citrus Shrimp Salad

Bright, zesty, and full of flavor, this Citrus Shrimp Salad is a refreshing dish perfect for warm days or when you're in the mood for something light yet satisfying. The combination of juicy shrimp, crisp greens, and tangy citrus dressing makes this salad a must-try.

- Prep Time: 10 minutes
- Cook Time: 10 minutes
- Total Time: 20 minutes
- Servings: 2

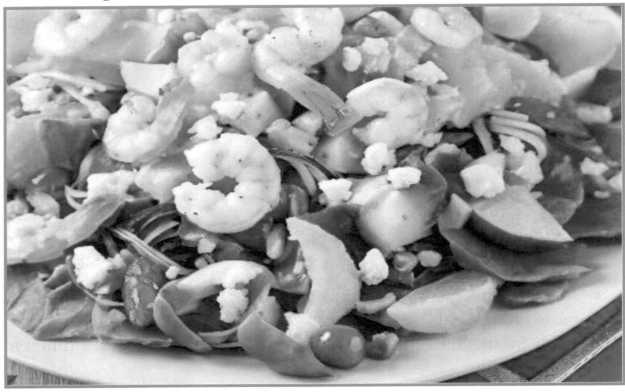

Ingredients:

- 12 large shrimp, peeled and deveined
- 1 teaspoon olive oil
- 1 teaspoon garlic powder
- Salt and pepper to taste
- 4 cups mixed greens (spinach, arugula, or spring mix)
- 1 orange, peeled and segmented
- 1/2 avocado, sliced
- 1/4 cup red onion, thinly sliced
- 1 tablespoon chopped fresh mint or cilantro (optional)

Dressing:

- 2 tablespoons fresh orange juice
- 1 tablespoon lemon juice
- 1 teaspoon Dijon mustard
- 1 teaspoon honey
- 1 teaspoon olive oil
- Salt and pepper to taste

Instructions:

1. Cook the Shrimp: Heat 1 teaspoon of olive oil in a skillet over medium heat. Season the shrimp with garlic powder, salt, and pepper. Cook for 2-3 minutes per side, or until the shrimp turn pink and opaque. Remove from heat and let cool slightly.
2. Make the Dressing: In a small bowl, whisk together the orange juice, lemon juice, Dijon mustard, honey, olive oil, salt, and pepper until smooth and well combined.
3. Assemble the Salad: Arrange the mixed greens on two plates or in bowls. Top with orange segments, avocado slices, red onion, and cooked shrimp.
4. Add Dressing: Drizzle the citrus dressing over the salad and toss lightly to coat. Garnish with fresh mint or cilantro if desired.
5. Serve and Enjoy: Serve immediately for the freshest flavors.

Nutrition Information (per serving):

- Calories: 250

- Protein: 20g
- Carbohydrates: 15g
- Fat: 12g
- Fiber: 5g
- Sugar: 6g

Points Value: 5 WW Points per serving

Tips & Variations:

- Protein Swap: Substitute shrimp with grilled chicken or tofu for a different take on this salad.
- Extra Crunch: Add a handful of sliced almonds or sunflower seeds for added texture.
- Meal Prep: Keep the dressing separate until ready to serve to maintain the salad's crispness.

This Citrus Shrimp Salad is a bright and refreshing way to enjoy a high-protein, low-Points meal. With its vibrant flavors and satisfying textures, it's sure to become a favorite in your healthy eating repertoire.

Mediterranean Chickpea Salad

Hearty and bursting with Mediterranean flavors, this Mediterranean Chickpea Salad is a simple yet satisfying dish perfect for lunch or as a side at your next gathering. It's packed with fresh vegetables, tangy feta, and wholesome chickpeas for a filling and nutritious meal.

- Prep Time: 15 minutes
- Cook Time: 0 minutes
- Total Time: 15 minutes
- Servings: 4

Ingredients:

- 1 can (15 ounces) chickpeas, drained and rinsed
- 1 cup cherry tomatoes, halved
- 1 cup cucumber, diced
- 1/2 cup red bell pepper, diced

- 1/4 cup red onion, finely chopped
- 1/4 cup Kalamata olives, halved
- 1/4 cup crumbled feta cheese
- 2 tablespoons chopped fresh parsley
- 2 tablespoons olive oil
- 1 tablespoon red wine vinegar
- 1 teaspoon lemon juice
- 1 teaspoon dried oregano
- Salt and pepper to taste

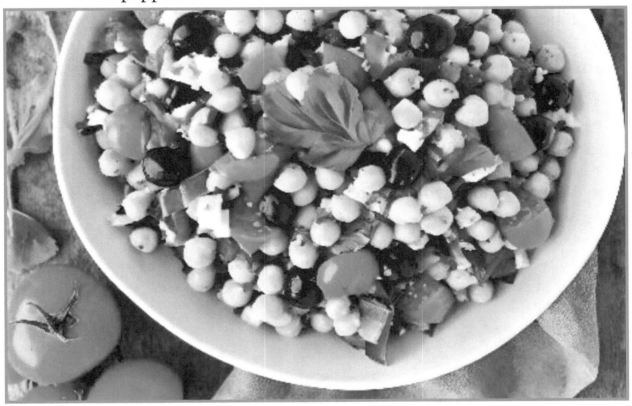

Instructions:

1. Prepare the Ingredients: Drain and rinse the chickpeas. Chop all the vegetables and parsley.
2. Make the Dressing: In a small bowl, whisk together the olive oil, red wine vinegar, lemon juice, oregano, salt, and pepper.
3. Combine Ingredients: In a large mixing bowl, combine the chickpeas, cherry tomatoes, cucumber, red bell pepper, red onion, olives, feta cheese, and parsley.

4. Add the Dressing: Pour the dressing over the salad and toss until everything is evenly coated.
5. Serve and Enjoy: Serve immediately or let the salad sit in the fridge for 30 minutes to allow the flavors to meld together.

Nutrition Information (per serving):

- Calories: 200
- Protein: 6g
- Carbohydrates: 22g
- Fat: 9g
- Fiber: 6g
- Sugar: 3g

Points Value: 4 WW Points per serving

Tips & Variations:

- Extra Protein: Add grilled chicken or canned tuna to turn this salad into a heartier meal.
- Herb Swap: Substitute parsley with basil or dill for a new flavor twist.
- Vegan Option: Omit the feta cheese or replace it with a plant-based alternative.

This Mediterranean Chickpea Salad combines vibrant flavors with wholesome ingredients for a salad that's as satisfying as it is nutritious. Whether served as a main course or a side, it's a dish that's sure to impress and nourish.

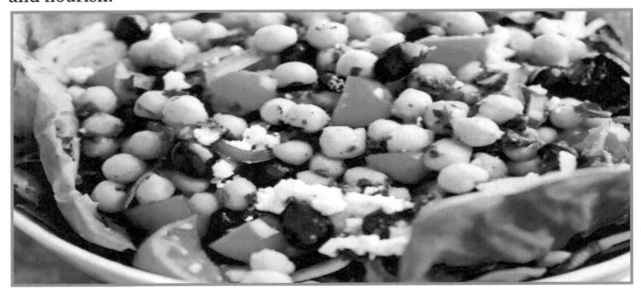

Chapter 3: Soups & Starters

Soups and starters are the heartwarming beginnings of any meal. They're versatile, satisfying, and packed with flavor. Whether you're craving a light, fresh option or a hearty, filling bowl, these recipes offer something for everyone. Perfect as appetizers or stand-alone meals, these soups and starters are designed to fit seamlessly into your Weight Watchers plan.

Tomato Basil Soup

This classic Tomato Basil Soup is a timeless favorite, made with simple, wholesome ingredients and bursting with fresh flavors. It's creamy without the cream, light without sacrificing taste, and perfect for a cozy night in or a light lunch.

- Prep Time: 10 minutes
- Cook Time: 30 minutes
- Total Time: 40 minutes
- Servings: 4

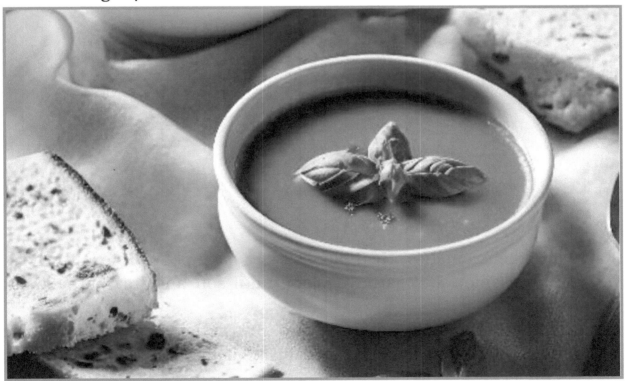

Ingredients:

- 1 tablespoon olive oil
- 1 small onion, finely chopped
- 2 cloves garlic, minced
- 1 can (28 ounces) crushed tomatoes
- 2 cups low-sodium vegetable broth
- 1 teaspoon dried oregano
- 1 teaspoon sugar (optional, to balance acidity)
- Salt and pepper to taste
- 1/4 cup fresh basil leaves, chopped
- Optional: 2 tablespoons grated Parmesan cheese for garnish

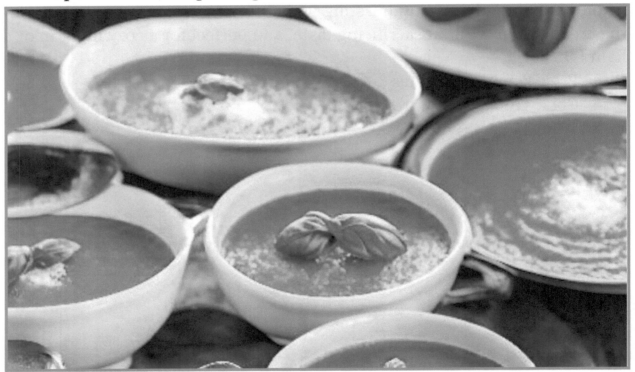

Instructions:

1. Sauté the Aromatics: Heat olive oil in a large pot over medium heat. Add the onion and garlic, cooking until soft and fragrant, about 5 minutes.
2. Add the Tomatoes and Broth: Stir in the crushed tomatoes, vegetable broth, oregano, sugar (if using), salt, and pepper. Bring the mixture to a simmer.

3. Cook the Soup: Cover and simmer for 20 minutes, stirring occasionally to let the flavors meld.
4. Blend to Perfection: Use an immersion blender to puree the soup until smooth. Alternatively, carefully transfer the soup to a blender and blend in batches.
5. Add the Basil: Stir in the fresh basil just before serving to retain its bright flavor.
6. Serve and Enjoy: Ladle the soup into bowls and garnish with grated Parmesan cheese, if desired.

Nutrition Information (per serving):

- Calories: 120
- Protein: 3g
- Carbohydrates: 16g
- Fat: 5g
- Fiber: 4g
- Sugar: 8g

Points Value: 3 WW Points per serving

Tips & Variations:

- Creamy Option: Add 1/4 cup of unsweetened almond milk for a creamier texture without adding many Points.
- Spicy Kick: Add a pinch of red pepper flakes for some heat.
- Meal Pairing: Pair with a slice of whole-grain bread or a side salad for a more complete meal.

This Tomato Basil Soup is the perfect combination of fresh, tangy, and comforting flavors. Whether you're enjoying it as a starter or a light main dish, it's a classic recipe that never goes out of style.

Spicy Lentil Stew

Hearty, nutritious, and packed with flavor, this Spicy Lentil Stew is the ultimate comfort food. It's high in fiber and protein, making it a filling option for a main meal or a satisfying starter on cooler days.

- Prep Time: 10 minutes

- Cook Time: 35 minutes
- Total Time: 45 minutes
- Servings: 4

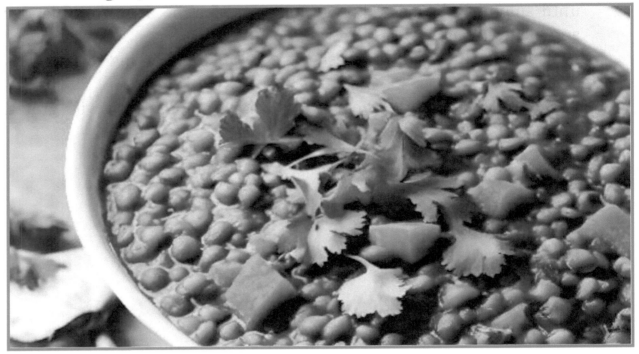

Ingredients:
- 1 tablespoon olive oil
- 1 small onion, diced
- 2 carrots, diced
- 2 celery stalks, diced
- 2 cloves garlic, minced
- 1 teaspoon ground cumin
- 1/2 teaspoon smoked paprika
- 1/4 teaspoon cayenne pepper (adjust for spice level)
- 1 cup dried red lentils, rinsed
- 4 cups low-sodium vegetable broth
- 1 can (14.5 ounces) diced tomatoes
- 1/2 teaspoon salt, or to taste
- 1/4 teaspoon black pepper
- Juice of 1/2 lemon
- 2 tablespoons chopped fresh parsley for garnish

Instructions:

1. Sauté the Vegetables: Heat olive oil in a large pot over medium heat. Add the onion, carrots, and celery, cooking until softened, about 5 minutes. Add the garlic and cook for another minute.
2. Add Spices and Lentils: Stir in the cumin, smoked paprika, and cayenne pepper. Add the lentils and toss to coat in the spices.
3. Simmer the Stew: Pour in the vegetable broth and diced tomatoes. Bring the mixture to a boil, then reduce the heat to low. Cover and simmer for 30 minutes, or until the lentils are tender.
4. Finish with Lemon: Stir in the lemon juice and adjust seasoning with salt and pepper to taste.
5. Serve and Garnish: Ladle the stew into bowls and garnish with fresh parsley. Serve hot.

Nutrition Information (per serving):

- Calories: 200
- Protein: 12g
- Carbohydrates: 30g
- Fat: 4g
- Fiber: 12g
- Sugar: 6g

Points Value: 4 WW Points per serving

Tips & Variations:

- Add Greens: Stir in a handful of fresh spinach or kale during the last 5 minutes of cooking for extra nutrients.
- Milder Option: Reduce or omit the cayenne pepper if you prefer a less spicy stew.
- Make It Ahead: This stew tastes even better the next day, making it perfect for meal prep.

This Spicy Lentil Stew is a comforting dish that delivers warmth and nutrition in every bite. With its rich, bold flavors and hearty texture, it's a recipe that's sure to become a household favorite.

Zucchini Crisps

Light, crispy, and utterly irresistible, these Zucchini Crisps are a healthier alternative to chips or fries. Perfect as an appetizer or a snack, they're baked to golden perfection and seasoned just right.

- Prep Time: 10 minutes
- Cook Time: 20 minutes
- Total Time: 30 minutes
- Servings: 4

Ingredients:

- 2 medium zucchinis, thinly sliced into rounds
- 1/2 cup whole wheat breadcrumbs
- 1/4 cup grated Parmesan cheese
- 1 teaspoon garlic powder
- 1 teaspoon dried Italian seasoning
- 1/2 teaspoon salt
- 1/4 teaspoon black pepper
- 1 large egg, beaten
- Cooking spray

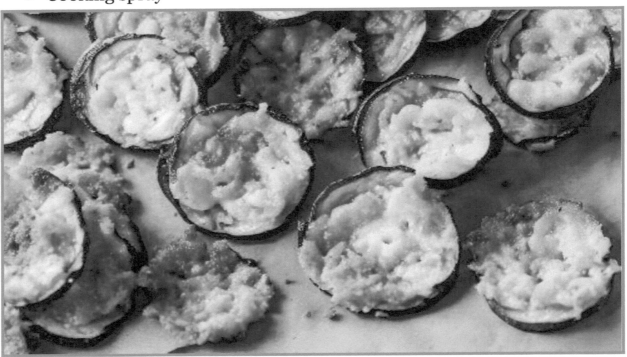

Instructions:

1. Preheat the Oven: Preheat your oven to 425°F (220°C). Line a baking sheet with parchment paper or a silicone baking mat and lightly spray with cooking spray.
2. Prepare the Breading Mixture: In a shallow bowl, combine the breadcrumbs, Parmesan cheese, garlic powder, Italian seasoning, salt, and pepper.
3. Coat the Zucchini: Dip each zucchini slice into the beaten egg, then coat it in the breadcrumb mixture, pressing gently to adhere.
4. Arrange and Bake: Place the coated zucchini slices in a single layer on the prepared baking sheet. Lightly spray the tops with cooking spray. Bake for 20 minutes, flipping halfway through, until golden and crispy.
5. Serve and Enjoy: Allow to cool slightly before serving with your favorite low-fat dipping sauce or marinara.

Nutrition Information (per serving):

- Calories: 110
- Protein: 5g
- Carbohydrates: 12g
- Fat: 5g
- Fiber: 2g
- Sugar: 2g

Points Value: 3 WW Points per serving

Tips & Variations:

- Gluten-Free Option: Use gluten-free breadcrumbs to make this dish suitable for gluten-free diets.
- Extra Crunch: Add a tablespoon of panko breadcrumbs for added crispiness.
- Spice It Up: Add a pinch of cayenne or smoked paprika to the breading mixture for a kick.

These Zucchini Crisps are proof that healthy snacks can still satisfy your cravings. Light and full of flavor, they're an easy way to enjoy your veggies while indulging in a crispy bite.

Cauliflower Buffalo Bites

These Cauliflower Buffalo Bites are the ultimate guilt-free snack or appetizer. With their spicy kick and tender texture, they're a healthier alternative to traditional wings that will have everyone coming back for more.

- Prep Time: 10 minutes
- Cook Time: 30 minutes
- Total Time: 40 minutes
- Servings: 4

Ingredients:

- 1 medium head of cauliflower, cut into bite-sized florets
- 1/2 cup whole wheat flour
- 1/2 cup unsweetened almond milk
- 1 teaspoon garlic powder
- 1/2 teaspoon smoked paprika
- 1/4 teaspoon salt
- 1/4 teaspoon black pepper
- 1/2 cup hot sauce (such as Frank's RedHot)
- 1 tablespoon melted butter or olive oil

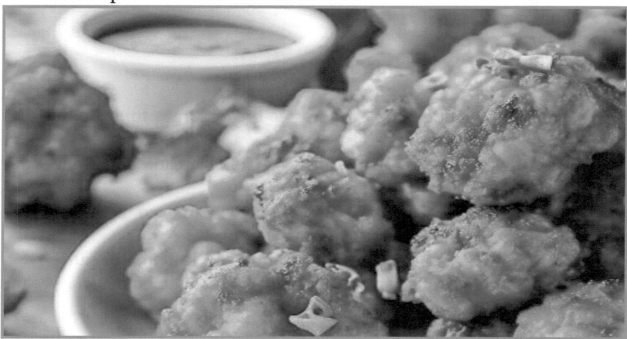

Instructions:

1. Preheat the Oven: Preheat your oven to 450°F (230°C). Line a baking sheet with parchment paper or a silicone mat.
2. Prepare the Batter: In a large bowl, whisk together the flour, almond milk, garlic powder, smoked paprika, salt, and pepper until smooth.
3. Coat the Cauliflower: Dip each cauliflower floret into the batter, shaking off any excess, and place it on the prepared baking sheet.
4. Bake Until Crisp: Bake for 20 minutes, flipping halfway through, until the cauliflower is lightly browned and crispy.
5. Toss in Sauce: In a small bowl, mix the hot sauce with melted butter or olive oil. Remove the cauliflower from the oven and toss the florets in the sauce until evenly coated.
6. Finish Baking: Return the cauliflower to the baking sheet and bake for an additional 10 minutes, or until the sauce is slightly caramelized.
7. Serve and Enjoy: Serve warm with a side of low-fat ranch or blue cheese dressing for dipping.

Nutrition Information (per serving):

- Calories: 120
- Protein: 3g
- Carbohydrates: 15g
- Fat: 5g
- Fiber: 3g
- Sugar: 2g

Points Value: 4 WW Points per serving

Tips & Variations:

- Milder Option: Adjust the amount of hot sauce for a less spicy version.
- Air Fryer Option: Cook the cauliflower in an air fryer at 400°F for 15-20 minutes for an even crispier texture.
- Dipping Sauce: Serve with a side of Greek yogurt mixed with a little garlic and dill for a healthier alternative to ranch.

These Cauliflower Buffalo Bites are a flavorful, satisfying option that packs a punch without the added guilt. Perfect for game day, parties, or a spicy snack, they're sure to become a favorite in your healthy recipe lineup.

Chapter 4: Proteins

Proteins are the cornerstone of a balanced diet, providing the fuel you need to stay energized throughout the day. These recipes highlight lean and flavorful options that are easy to prepare and packed with nutrients, making them perfect for any meal.

Herb-Crusted Salmon

This Herb-Crusted Salmon is a show-stopping dish that's as simple as it is delicious. The crispy herb coating perfectly complements the tender, flaky salmon, making it a protein-packed meal you'll turn to time and again.

- Prep Time: 10 minutes
- Cook Time: 15 minutes
- Total Time: 25 minutes
- Servings: 4

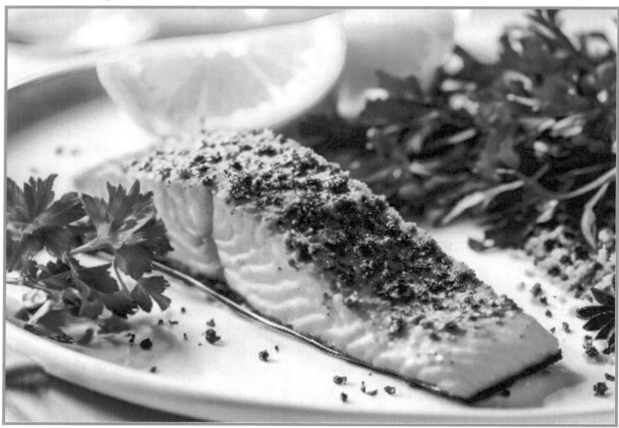

Ingredients:

- 4 salmon fillets (4-5 ounces each)
- 1 tablespoon olive oil
- 1/2 cup whole wheat breadcrumbs
- 1/4 cup grated Parmesan cheese
- 2 tablespoons fresh parsley, chopped
- 1 tablespoon fresh dill, chopped
- 1 teaspoon lemon zest
- 1 clove garlic, minced
- 1/4 teaspoon salt
- 1/4 teaspoon black pepper
- Lemon wedges, for serving

Instructions:

1. Preheat the Oven: Preheat your oven to 400°F (200°C). Line a baking sheet with parchment paper or lightly grease it.
2. Prepare the Herb Mixture: In a small bowl, mix the breadcrumbs, Parmesan cheese, parsley, dill, lemon zest, garlic, salt, and pepper.
3. Brush the Salmon: Pat the salmon fillets dry with a paper towel and brush the tops lightly with olive oil.
4. Add the Herb Crust: Press the breadcrumb mixture onto the tops of the salmon fillets, ensuring an even coating.
5. Bake the Salmon: Place the fillets on the prepared baking sheet and bake for 12-15 minutes, or until the salmon flakes easily with a fork and the crust is golden brown.
6. Serve and Enjoy: Serve hot with lemon wedges for a bright, fresh finish.

Nutrition Information (per serving):

- Calories: 280
- Protein: 30g
- Carbohydrates: 6g
- Fat: 16g
- Fiber: 1g
- Sugar: 0g

Points Value: 5 WW Points per serving

Tips & Variations:

- No Breadcrumbs? Substitute with almond flour for a gluten-free option.
- Add Veggies: Roast asparagus or broccoli alongside the salmon for a complete meal.
- Air Fryer Option: Cook in an air fryer at 375°F for 10-12 minutes for extra crispiness.

This Herb-Crusted Salmon is a perfect balance of crispy, savory, and fresh. It's an elegant dish that's easy enough for weeknights but impressive enough for entertaining.

Turkey Veggie Meatballs

These Turkey Veggie Meatballs are a healthier take on the classic comfort food. Packed with lean turkey and nutrient-rich vegetables, they're juicy, flavorful, and perfect for meal prep or family dinners.

- Prep Time: 15 minutes
- Cook Time: 20 minutes
- Total Time: 35 minutes
- Servings: 4 (12 meatballs)

Ingredients:

- 1 pound ground turkey (93% lean)
- 1/2 cup zucchini, grated
- 1/2 cup carrot, grated
- 1/4 cup whole wheat breadcrumbs
- 1 egg, lightly beaten
- 2 tablespoons fresh parsley, chopped
- 1 teaspoon garlic powder
- 1 teaspoon onion powder
- 1/2 teaspoon salt
- 1/4 teaspoon black pepper
- Cooking spray

Instructions:

1. Preheat the Oven: Preheat your oven to 375°F (190°C). Line a baking sheet with parchment paper and lightly spray with cooking spray.

2. Prepare the Mixture: In a large bowl, combine the ground turkey, grated zucchini, grated carrot, breadcrumbs, egg, parsley, garlic powder, onion powder, salt, and pepper. Mix gently until all ingredients are evenly distributed.

3. Shape the Meatballs: Using your hands or a cookie scoop, form the mixture into 12 evenly sized meatballs. Place them on the prepared baking sheet.

4. Bake the Meatballs: Bake for 18-20 minutes, or until the meatballs are cooked through and reach an internal temperature of 165°F (74°C).

5. Serve and Enjoy: Serve the meatballs with marinara sauce, over zucchini noodles, or alongside a salad for a balanced meal.

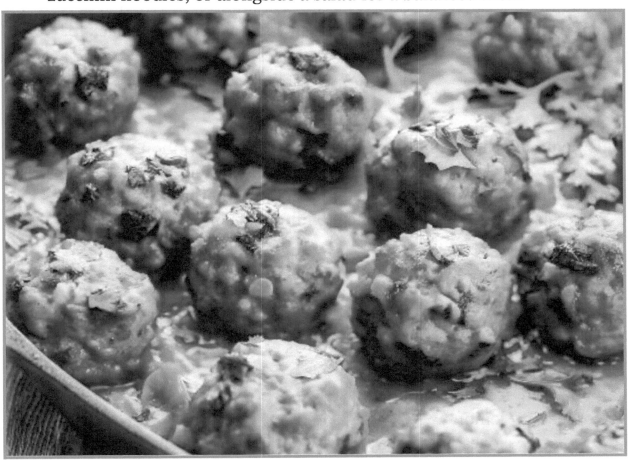

Nutrition Information (per serving):

- Calories: 200
- Protein: 25g
- Carbohydrates: 8g
- Fat: 8g
- Fiber: 2g
- Sugar: 2g

Points Value: 4 WW Points per serving

Tips & Variations:

- Meal Prep: These meatballs freeze well. Simply cool completely, store in an airtight container, and freeze for up to three months.
- Add Heat: Incorporate a pinch of red pepper flakes for a spicy kick.
- Sauce Ideas: Pair with a teriyaki glaze or a light tzatziki for variety.

These Turkey Veggie Meatballs are packed with flavor and nutrients, making them a satisfying and versatile protein option. Whether served solo or with your favorite sides, they're a dish you'll keep coming back to.

Lemon Grilled Chicken

This Lemon Grilled Chicken is a zesty and flavorful option that's perfect for meal prep, weeknight dinners, or even a summer barbecue. The bright lemon marinade infuses the chicken with tangy, herbaceous goodness.

- Prep Time: 10 minutes (plus 30 minutes marinating time)
- Cook Time: 15 minutes
- Total Time: 55 minutes
- Servings: 4

Ingredients:

- 4 boneless, skinless chicken breasts (4-5 ounces each)
- 1/4 cup olive oil
- 1/4 cup fresh lemon juice
- Zest of 1 lemon
- 3 garlic cloves, minced

- 1 teaspoon dried oregano
- 1/2 teaspoon salt
- 1/4 teaspoon black pepper
- Fresh parsley, chopped (for garnish)

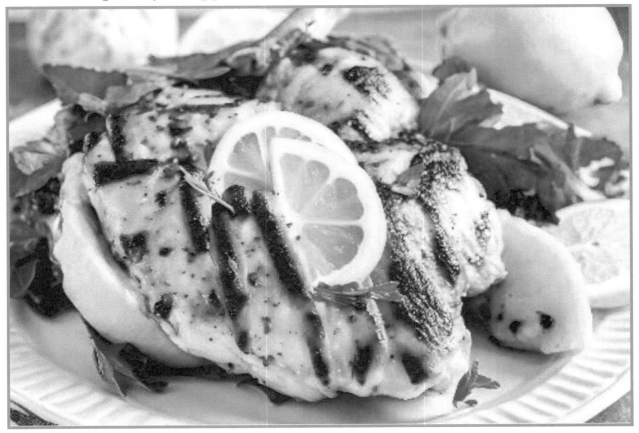

Instructions:

1. Prepare the Marinade: In a small bowl, whisk together the olive oil, lemon juice, lemon zest, garlic, oregano, salt, and pepper.
2. Marinate the Chicken: Place the chicken breasts in a shallow dish or a resealable plastic bag. Pour the marinade over the chicken, ensuring it's well-coated. Cover and refrigerate for at least 30 minutes or up to 4 hours for deeper flavor.
3. Preheat the Grill: Preheat your grill or grill pan over medium-high heat. Lightly oil the grates to prevent sticking.
4. Grill the Chicken: Remove the chicken from the marinade and discard the excess. Grill the chicken for 6-8 minutes per side, or until fully cooked and the internal temperature reaches 165°F (74°C).

5. Serve and Garnish: Transfer the chicken to a serving plate, garnish with fresh parsley, and serve with lemon wedges.

Nutrition Information (per serving):

- Calories: 200
- Protein: 30g
- Carbohydrates: 1g
- Fat: 8g
- Fiber: 0g
- Sugar: 0g

Points Value: 4 WW Points per serving

Tips & Variations:

- Oven Option: If you don't have a grill, bake the chicken at 400°F for 20-25 minutes.
- Add Spice: For a spicy kick, add a pinch of red pepper flakes to the marinade.
- Serve Ideas: Pair with roasted vegetables, a side salad, or quinoa for a balanced meal.

This Lemon Grilled Chicken is a light and flavorful dish that's as versatile as it is delicious. Its zesty flavors and juicy texture make it a go-to option for any occasion.

Baked Teriyaki Tofu

This Baked Teriyaki Tofu is a plant-based protein option that's packed with umami flavors. Crispy on the outside and tender on the inside, it's perfect for serving over rice, in a stir-fry, or as a standalone dish.

- Prep Time: 10 minutes
- Cook Time: 30 minutes
- Total Time: 40 minutes
- Servings: 4

Ingredients:

- 1 block (14 ounces) firm tofu, pressed and cut into cubes
- 2 tablespoons cornstarch

- Cooking spray

Teriyaki Sauce:
- 1/4 cup low-sodium soy sauce
- 2 tablespoons honey or maple syrup
- 1 tablespoon rice vinegar
- 1 teaspoon sesame oil
- 1 teaspoon grated fresh ginger
- 1 clove garlic, minced
- 1 teaspoon cornstarch mixed with 2 teaspoons water

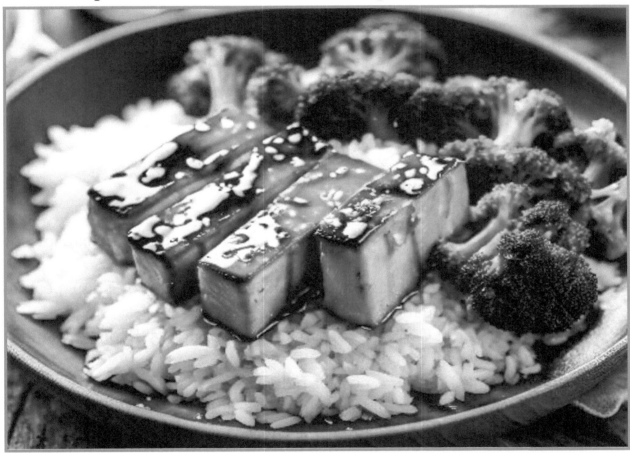

Instructions:

1. Preheat the Oven: Preheat your oven to 400°F (200°C). Line a baking sheet with parchment paper and lightly spray with cooking spray.
2. Prepare the Tofu: Toss the tofu cubes with cornstarch until evenly coated. Arrange the cubes in a single layer on the baking sheet and lightly spray the tops with cooking spray.

3. Bake the Tofu: Bake for 25-30 minutes, flipping halfway through, until the tofu is golden and crispy.
4. Make the Teriyaki Sauce: In a small saucepan, combine the soy sauce, honey or maple syrup, rice vinegar, sesame oil, ginger, and garlic. Bring to a simmer over medium heat. Stir in the cornstarch slurry and cook until the sauce thickens, about 1-2 minutes.
5. Combine and Serve: Toss the baked tofu in the teriyaki sauce until fully coated. Serve over rice or steamed vegetables and garnish with sesame seeds or green onions if desired.

Nutrition Information (per serving):Ll

- Calories: 180
- Protein: 10g
- Carbohydrates: 15g
- Fat: 8g
- Fiber: 1g
- Sugar: 5g

Points Value: 4 WW Points per serving

Tips & Variations:

- Gluten-Free Option: Use tamari or coconut aminos instead of soy sauce.
- Extra Veggies: Add roasted broccoli, bell peppers, or snap peas to make it a complete meal.
- Air Fryer Option: Cook the tofu in an air fryer at 375°F for 15 minutes, shaking halfway through.

This Baked Teriyaki Tofu is a perfect balance of crispy and savory, with a homemade teriyaki sauce that's simply irresistible. It's a versatile and satisfying dish for plant-based and meat-eaters alike.

Chapter 5: Main Dishes

Main dishes are the centerpiece of any meal, and these recipes deliver bold flavors, balanced nutrition, and ease of preparation. Whether you're in the mood for a quick stir-fry or a hearty pasta dish, these options will keep you full and satisfied without compromising your health goals

Veggie Stir-Fry

This Veggie Stir-Fry is a vibrant and flavorful dish that's ready in minutes. Packed with colorful vegetables and tossed in a savory sauce, it's a versatile recipe that can stand alone or pair beautifully with your favorite protein.

- Prep Time: 10 minutes
- Cook Time: 15 minutes
- Total Time: 25 minutes
- Servings: 4

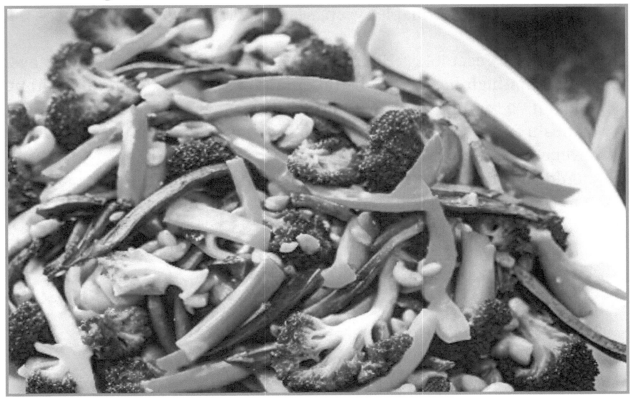

Ingredients:

- 1 tablespoon olive oil
- 1 small onion, sliced
- 2 cloves garlic, minced
- 1 cup broccoli florets
- 1 cup bell peppers, sliced
- 1 cup snap peas
- 1 cup sliced mushrooms
- 1 medium zucchini, sliced
- 1/4 cup low-sodium soy sauce
- 1 tablespoon rice vinegar
- 1 tablespoon honey or maple syrup
- 1 teaspoon sesame oil
- 1 teaspoon cornstarch mixed with 2 teaspoons water
- Sesame seeds and green onions for garnish

Instructions:

1. Prepare the Sauce: In a small bowl, whisk together the soy sauce, rice vinegar, honey or maple syrup, sesame oil, and cornstarch slurry. Set aside.
2. Cook the Vegetables: Heat the olive oil in a large skillet or wok over medium-high heat. Add the onion and garlic, cooking until fragrant, about 2 minutes. Add the broccoli, bell peppers, snap peas, mushrooms, and zucchini. Stir-fry for 8-10 minutes until the vegetables are tender but still crisp.
3. Add the Sauce: Pour the prepared sauce over the vegetables and toss to coat evenly. Cook for an additional 2-3 minutes, allowing the sauce to thicken slightly.
4. Serve and Garnish: Serve the stir-fry immediately, garnished with sesame seeds and green onions if desired.

Nutrition Information (per serving):

- Calories: 120
- Protein: 4g
- Carbohydrates: 15g

- Fat: 5g
- Fiber: 4g
- Sugar: 6g

Points Value: 3 WW Points per serving

Tips & Variations:

- Add Protein: Toss in tofu, shrimp, or grilled chicken for a more filling meal.
- Spicy Kick: Add red pepper flakes or sriracha to the sauce for a spicy twist.
- Serve With: Pair with brown rice, quinoa, or cauliflower rice for a complete meal.

This Veggie Stir-Fry is a fast and flavorful way to pack your plate with colorful vegetables. It's perfect for busy nights or when you're craving a light yet satisfying meal.

Whole Wheat Pasta Primavera

This Whole Wheat Pasta Primavera is a classic Italian-inspired dish, loaded with fresh vegetables and tossed in a light garlic and olive oil sauce. It's a hearty yet wholesome option for pasta lovers.

- Prep Time: 10 minutes
- Cook Time: 20 minutes
- Total Time: 30 minutes
- Servings: 4

Ingredients:

- 8 ounces whole wheat pasta (spaghetti, penne, or your choice)
- 1 tablespoon olive oil
- 2 cloves garlic, minced
- 1 cup cherry tomatoes, halved
- 1 cup zucchini, diced
- 1 cup yellow squash, diced
- 1 cup broccoli florets
- 1/2 cup bell peppers, diced

- 1/4 cup grated Parmesan cheese
- 1/4 cup fresh basil, chopped
- Salt and pepper to taste
- Lemon wedges for serving

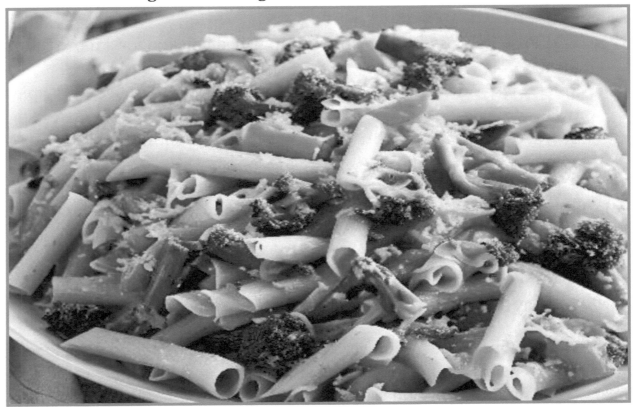

Instructions:

1. Cook the Pasta: Bring a large pot of salted water to a boil. Cook the pasta according to package instructions until al dente. Drain and set aside.
2. Sauté the Vegetables: In a large skillet, heat the olive oil over medium heat. Add the garlic and cook until fragrant, about 1 minute. Add the cherry tomatoes, zucchini, yellow squash, broccoli, and bell peppers. Sauté for 8-10 minutes, or until the vegetables are tender.
3. Combine Pasta and Vegetables: Add the cooked pasta to the skillet with the vegetables. Toss to combine and heat through.
4. Add Parmesan and Basil: Remove from heat and sprinkle with grated Parmesan cheese and fresh basil. Season with salt and pepper to taste.

5. Serve and Garnish: Serve warm with a squeeze of fresh lemon juice for brightness.

Nutrition Information (per serving):

- Calories: 300
- Protein: 10g
- Carbohydrates: 50g
- Fat: 8g
- Fiber: 7g
- Sugar: 6g

Points Value: 7 WW Points per serving

Tips & Variations:

- Creamy Option: Add a dollop of low-fat ricotta or a splash of almond milk for a creamy twist.
- Add Protein: Include grilled chicken, shrimp, or chickpeas for a protein boost.
- Extra Herbs: Garnish with parsley or oregano for additional flavor.

This Whole Wheat Pasta Primavera is a hearty yet healthy dish that brings together fresh vegetables and classic Italian flavors. It's perfect for a comforting meal that doesn't derail your goals.

Stuffed Bell Peppers

These Stuffed Bell Peppers are a colorful, nutrient-packed dish that's as beautiful as it is delicious. Loaded with a savory filling of lean protein, whole grains, and vegetables, they're a complete meal in one.

- Prep Time: 15 minutes
- Cook Time: 35 minutes
- Total Time: 50 minutes
- Servings: 4

Ingredients:

- 4 large bell peppers (any color)
- 1/2 pound ground turkey or lean ground beef

- 1/2 cup cooked quinoa or brown rice
- 1/2 cup diced tomatoes (canned or fresh)
- 1/2 cup diced onion
- 1/2 cup shredded mozzarella cheese (reduced-fat)
- 2 tablespoons tomato paste
- 1 teaspoon garlic powder
- 1 teaspoon Italian seasoning
- 1/2 teaspoon salt
- 1/4 teaspoon black pepper
- Fresh parsley, chopped (for garnish)

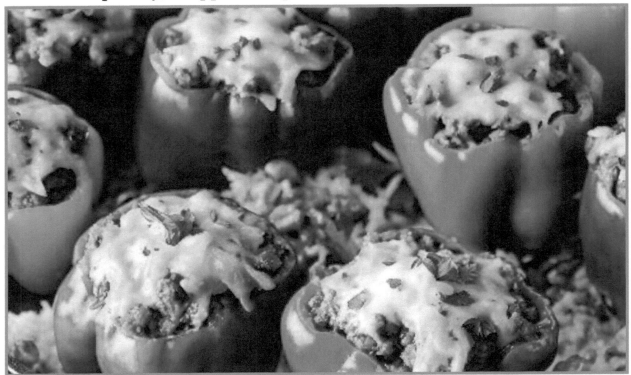

Instructions:

1. Preheat the Oven: Preheat your oven to 375°F (190°C). Lightly grease a baking dish.
2. Prepare the Peppers: Cut the tops off the bell peppers and remove the seeds and membranes. Place them in the baking dish, standing upright.
3. Cook the Filling: Heat a skillet over medium heat. Add the ground turkey or beef and diced onion, cooking until the meat is browned.

Stir in the cooked quinoa or brown rice, diced tomatoes, tomato paste, garlic powder, Italian seasoning, salt, and pepper. Cook for 3-5 minutes to combine the flavors.

4. Stuff the Peppers: Spoon the filling into each bell pepper, packing it tightly. Top each pepper with shredded mozzarella cheese.
5. Bake: Cover the dish with aluminum foil and bake for 25 minutes. Remove the foil and bake for an additional 10 minutes, or until the cheese is melted and bubbly.
6. Serve and Garnish: Serve warm, garnished with fresh parsley.

Nutrition Information (per serving):

- Calories: 250
- Protein: 20g
- Carbohydrates: 20g
- Fat: 9g
- Fiber: 4g
- Sugar: 6g

Points Value: 5 WW Points per serving

Tips & Variations:

- Vegetarian Option: Replace the meat with black beans or lentils for a plant-based version.
- Spicy Kick: Add red pepper flakes or diced jalapeños to the filling for extra heat.
- Meal Prep: These peppers reheat beautifully, making them perfect for leftovers.

These Stuffed Bell Peppers are as satisfying as they are nutritious. They're a great way to enjoy a complete meal in a single dish while keeping things light and flavorful.

Light Eggplant Parmesan

This Light Eggplant Parmesan is a healthier take on the classic Italian dish. With layers of tender eggplant, tangy marinara, and melted cheese, it's a comforting, veggie-forward meal that satisfies without the heaviness.

- Prep Time: 15 minutes
- Cook Time: 40 minutes
- Total Time: 55 minutes
- Servings: 4

Ingredients:

- 2 medium eggplants, sliced into 1/4-inch rounds
- 1/2 cup whole wheat breadcrumbs
- 1/4 cup grated Parmesan cheese
- 1 teaspoon Italian seasoning
- 1/2 teaspoon garlic powder
- 1/2 teaspoon salt
- 1/4 teaspoon black pepper
- 1 large egg, beaten
- 1 1/2 cups marinara sauce (low-sugar)
- 1 cup shredded mozzarella cheese (reduced-fat)
- Fresh basil leaves (for garnish)

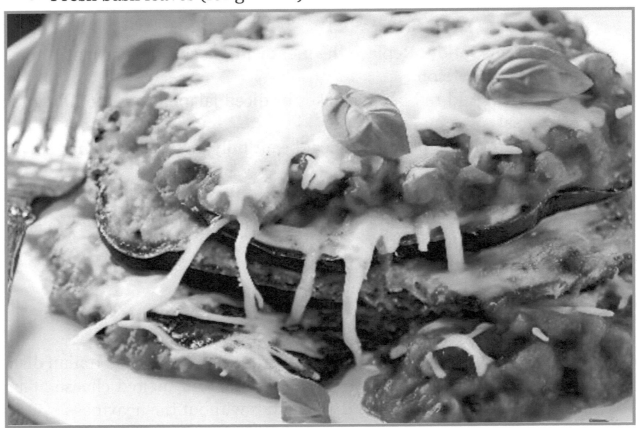

Instructions:

1. Preheat the Oven: Preheat your oven to 400°F (200°C). Line a baking sheet with parchment paper.
2. Prepare the Coating: In a shallow bowl, mix the breadcrumbs, Parmesan cheese, Italian seasoning, garlic powder, salt, and pepper.
3. Coat the Eggplant: Dip each eggplant slice into the beaten egg, then coat it in the breadcrumb mixture. Arrange the slices in a single layer on the prepared baking sheet.
4. Bake the Eggplant: Bake for 20 minutes, flipping halfway through, until golden and crispy.
5. Assemble the Dish: Spread a thin layer of marinara sauce in a 9x13-inch baking dish. Layer half the baked eggplant slices, top with half the marinara sauce, and sprinkle with half the mozzarella cheese. Repeat the layers.
6. Bake the Parmesan: Cover with foil and bake for 15 minutes. Remove the foil and bake for an additional 5 minutes, or until the cheese is melted and bubbly.
7. Serve and Garnish: Serve warm, garnished with fresh basil leaves.

Nutrition Information (per serving):

- Calories: 230
- Protein: 13g
- Carbohydrates: 20g
- Fat: 10g
- Fiber: 5g
- Sugar: 7g

Points Value: 6 WW Points per serving

Tips & Variations:

- Gluten-Free Option: Use gluten-free breadcrumbs for a gluten-free dish.
- Extra Veggies: Add a layer of sautéed spinach or mushrooms for added nutrition.
- Meal Prep: This dish reheats well, making it a great option for make-ahead meals.

Chapter 6: Sides

Sides are the perfect way to elevate any meal, adding texture, flavor, and variety. These simple yet delicious recipes are designed to pair well with a wide range of dishes while staying within your Weight Watchers Points budget.

Garlic Roasted Brussels

Crispy on the outside and tender on the inside, these Garlic Roasted Brussels are a flavorful and nutrient-packed side dish that will quickly become a favorite. The garlic adds a savory kick, while roasting brings out the natural sweetness of the Brussels sprouts.

- Prep Time: 10 minutes
- Cook Time: 25 minutes
- Total Time: 35 minutes
- Servings: 4

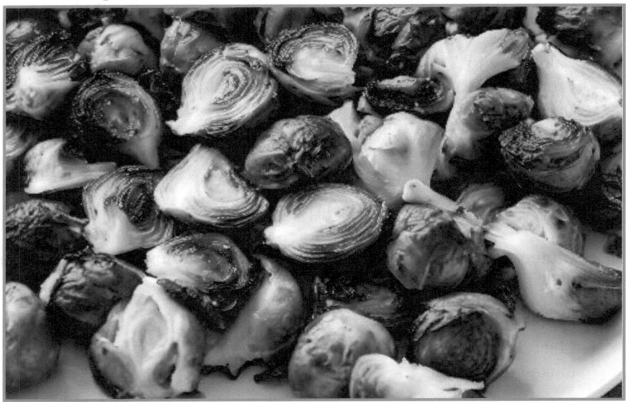

Ingredients:

- 1 pound Brussels sprouts, trimmed and halved
- 2 tablespoons olive oil
- 3 cloves garlic, minced
- 1/2 teaspoon salt
- 1/4 teaspoon black pepper
- Optional: 1 tablespoon grated Parmesan cheese or a squeeze of fresh lemon juice for garnish

Instructions:

1. Preheat the Oven: Preheat your oven to 400°F (200°C). Line a baking sheet with parchment paper.
2. Prepare the Brussels Sprouts: In a large bowl, toss the Brussels sprouts with olive oil, garlic, salt, and pepper until evenly coated.
3. Roast the Brussels Sprouts: Spread the Brussels sprouts in a single layer on the prepared baking sheet. Roast for 20-25 minutes, flipping halfway through, until the edges are golden and crispy.
4. Serve and Garnish: Serve hot, garnished with grated Parmesan or a squeeze of lemon juice if desired.

Nutrition Information (per serving):

- Calories: 100
- Protein: 3g
- Carbohydrates: 9g
- Fat: 7g
- Fiber: 3g
- Sugar: 2g

Points Value: 3 WW Points per serving

Tips & Variations:

- Add Crunch: Toss with sliced almonds or walnuts before roasting.
- Spicy Option: Add a pinch of red pepper flakes for a touch of heat.
- Extra Flavor: Drizzle with balsamic glaze just before serving.

Garlic Roasted Brussels are a simple yet impressive side dish that pairs beautifully with almost any main course. Their crispy edges and robust flavor make them a crowd-pleaser every time.

Sweet Potato Wedges

These Sweet Potato Wedges are the perfect balance of crispy and tender, with a touch of natural sweetness. They're seasoned to perfection and make a versatile side dish that complements everything from grilled proteins to hearty salads.

- Prep Time: 10 minutes
- Cook Time: 30 minutes
- Total Time: 40 minutes
- Servings: 4

Ingredients:

- 2 large sweet potatoes, cut into wedges
- 1 tablespoon olive oil
- 1 teaspoon paprika
- 1/2 teaspoon garlic powder
- 1/2 teaspoon salt
- 1/4 teaspoon black pepper
- Optional: Chopped fresh parsley for garnish

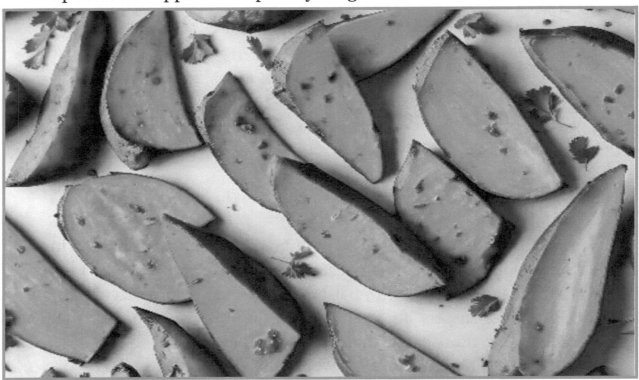

Instructions:

1. Preheat the Oven: Preheat your oven to 425°F (220°C). Line a baking sheet with parchment paper.
2. Season the Wedges: In a large bowl, toss the sweet potato wedges with olive oil, paprika, garlic powder, salt, and pepper until evenly coated.
3. Bake the Wedges: Arrange the wedges in a single layer on the prepared baking sheet. Bake for 25-30 minutes, flipping halfway through, until golden and tender.
4. Serve and Garnish: Serve hot, garnished with fresh parsley if desired.

Nutrition Information (per serving):

- Calories: 130
- Protein: 2g
- Carbohydrates: 23g
- Fat: 4g
- Fiber: 4g
- Sugar: 5g

Points Value: 4 WW Points per serving

Tips & Variations:

- Extra Crispy: For crispier wedges, soak the sweet potato slices in water for 30 minutes before baking and pat dry thoroughly.
- Spicy Kick: Sprinkle with cayenne pepper or chili powder for added heat.
- Dipping Sauce: Serve with a side of Greek yogurt mixed with a squeeze of lime and a dash of cumin for a refreshing dip.

These Sweet Potato Wedges are a healthier alternative to fries, with just the right balance of flavor and texture. They're a versatile side dish that's sure to please everyone at the table.

Cauliflower Mashed

This Cauliflower Mashed is a creamy, low-carb alternative to traditional mashed potatoes. It's rich, smooth, and packed with flavor, making it a comforting side dish without the extra calories or carbs.

- Prep Time: 10 minutes
- Cook Time: 15 minutes
- Total Time: 25 minutes
- Servings: 4

Ingredients:

- 1 medium head of cauliflower, cut into florets
- 2 tablespoons low-fat cream cheese
- 1 tablespoon unsalted butter
- 1 clove garlic, minced
- 1/4 cup grated Parmesan cheese
- 1/4 teaspoon salt
- 1/4 teaspoon black pepper
- Optional: Chopped fresh chives or parsley for garnish

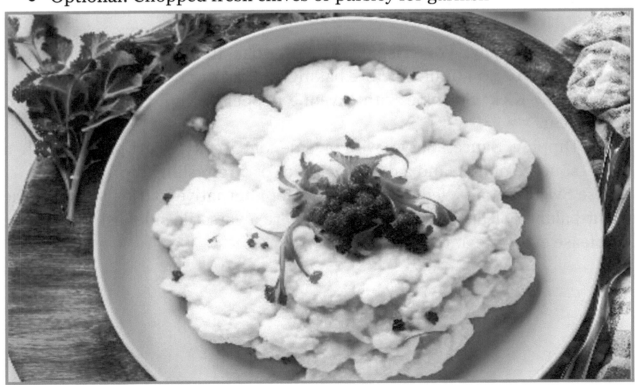

Instructions:

1. Steam the Cauliflower: In a large pot, steam the cauliflower florets until tender, about 10-12 minutes. Drain well and let cool slightly.
2. Blend the Cauliflower: In a food processor or blender, combine the steamed cauliflower, cream cheese, butter, garlic, Parmesan cheese, salt, and pepper. Blend until smooth and creamy.
3. Adjust Seasoning: Taste and adjust seasoning if needed. For a thicker consistency, blend less, leaving small chunks of cauliflower.
4. Serve and Garnish: Transfer to a serving bowl and garnish with fresh chives or parsley if desired. Serve warm.

Nutrition Information (per serving):

- Calories: 100
- Protein: 4g
- Carbohydrates: 6g
- Fat: 7g
- Fiber: 3g
- Sugar: 2g

Points Value: 3 WW Points per serving

Tips & Variations:

- Dairy-Free Option: Substitute the cream cheese and butter with unsweetened almond milk and olive oil for a dairy-free version.
- Extra Flavor: Add roasted garlic or a pinch of nutmeg for a unique twist.
- Meal Prep: Make ahead and reheat gently on the stovetop or in the microwave.

This Cauliflower Mashed is a creamy, satisfying side dish that's perfect for pairing with proteins or enjoying on its own. It's comfort food reimagined in a healthier way.

Herbed Quinoa Pilaf

This Herbed Quinoa Pilaf is a flavorful and nutrient-dense side dish that's perfect for adding a touch of elegance to your meals. Infused with fresh herbs and light seasonings, it's a versatile recipe that pairs well with a variety of proteins.

- Prep Time: 10 minutes
- Cook Time: 20 minutes
- Total Time: 30 minutes
- Servings: 4

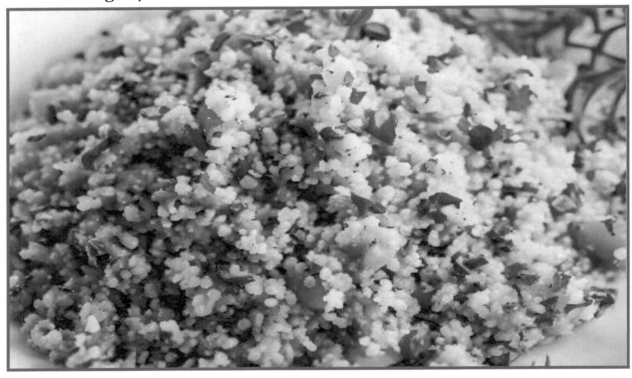

Ingredients:

- 1 cup quinoa, rinsed
- 2 cups low-sodium vegetable broth
- 1 tablespoon olive oil
- 1 small onion, finely chopped
- 1 clove garlic, minced
- 1/4 cup fresh parsley, chopped
- 1/4 cup fresh dill or cilantro, chopped

- Zest of 1 lemon
- Salt and pepper to taste
- Optional: Toasted almonds or pine nuts for garnish

Instructions:

1. Cook the Quinoa: In a medium saucepan, bring the vegetable broth to a boil. Add the rinsed quinoa, reduce the heat to low, cover, and simmer for 15 minutes, or until the quinoa is tender and the liquid is absorbed. Fluff with a fork and set aside.
2. Sauté the Aromatics: In a large skillet, heat the olive oil over medium heat. Add the onion and garlic, cooking until softened, about 3-4 minutes.
3. Combine Ingredients: Stir the cooked quinoa into the skillet with the onion and garlic. Add the parsley, dill, lemon zest, salt, and pepper. Mix until well combined and heated through.
4. Serve and Garnish: Transfer to a serving dish and garnish with toasted almonds or pine nuts if desired. Serve warm.

Nutrition Information (per serving):

- Calories: 180
- Protein: 6g
- Carbohydrates: 27g
- Fat: 5g
- Fiber: 3g
- Sugar: 1g

Points Value: 5 WW Points per serving

Tips & Variations:

- Add Veggies: Mix in sautéed mushrooms, spinach, or diced bell peppers for extra nutrition.
- Protein Boost: Add chickpeas or roasted chicken to make it a complete meal.
- Meal Prep: This pilaf keeps well in the fridge for up to three days, making it a great option for meal prep.

This Herbed Quinoa Pilaf is a light and flavorful side dish that brings a touch of sophistication to any meal. With its fresh herbs and citrusy notes, it's a perfect complement to a variety of main courses.

Chapter 7: Desserts

Desserts can be indulgent and healthy at the same time! These recipes are designed to satisfy your sweet tooth while staying within your Weight Watchers Points budget. With simple ingredients and easy preparation, these treats are as enjoyable to make as they are to eat.

Yogurt Berry Parfait

This Yogurt Berry Parfait is a simple yet elegant dessert that layers creamy yogurt, juicy berries, and crunchy granola for a delightful balance of flavors and textures. It's a versatile treat that's perfect for dessert, breakfast, or a snack.

- Prep Time: 5 minutes
- Cook Time: 0 minutes
- Total Time: 5 minutes
- Servings: 2

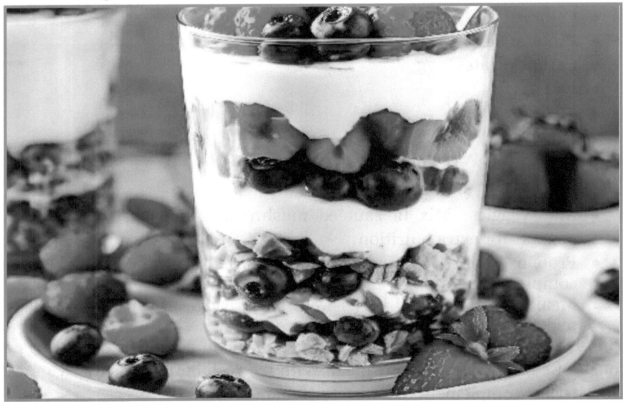

Ingredients:

- 1 cup non-fat Greek yogurt
- 1/2 cup mixed fresh berries (strawberries, blueberries, raspberries)
- 1/4 cup low-sugar granola
- 1 tablespoon honey or maple syrup (optional)
- 1 teaspoon chia seeds (optional)

Instructions:

Prepare the Ingredients: Wash and pat dry the fresh berries. Set aside.

1. Layer the Parfait: In a clear glass or dessert bowl, layer 1/4 cup of Greek yogurt at the bottom. Top with a layer of berries and a sprinkle of granola. Repeat the layers until the ingredients are used up.
2. Add Sweetener (Optional): Drizzle with honey or maple syrup for added sweetness if desired. Sprinkle with chia seeds for a nutritional boost.
3. Serve and Enjoy: Serve immediately for the freshest taste and crunch.

Nutrition Information (per serving):

- Calories: 120
- Protein: 10g
- Carbohydrates: 15g
- Fat: 2g
- Fiber: 3g
- Sugar: 8g

Points Value: 3 WW Points per serving

Tips & Variations:

- Dairy-Free Option: Use coconut or almond yogurt for a dairy-free version.
- Extra Crunch: Add a sprinkle of toasted nuts or seeds for added texture.
- Make Ahead: Assemble the parfait without the granola and store in the fridge. Add granola just before serving to maintain its crunch.

This Yogurt Berry Parfait is a quick and healthy dessert that's as beautiful as it is delicious. With its layers of creamy, sweet, and crunchy goodness, it's a treat you'll love to savor.

Dark Chocolate Chia Pudding

This Dark Chocolate Chia Pudding is rich, creamy, and full of chocolatey goodness. Made with nutrient-packed chia seeds, it's a guilt-free dessert that's also a great source of fiber and omega-3s.

- Prep Time: 5 minutes
- Cook Time: 0 minutes
- Chill Time: 4 hours (or overnight)
- Total Time: 4 hours 5 minutes
- Servings: 2

Ingredients:

- 1 cup unsweetened almond milk
- 2 tablespoons chia seeds
- 1 tablespoon unsweetened cocoa powder
- 1 tablespoon maple syrup or honey
- 1/2 teaspoon vanilla extract
- Optional toppings: Fresh berries, shaved dark chocolate, or a dollop of whipped cream

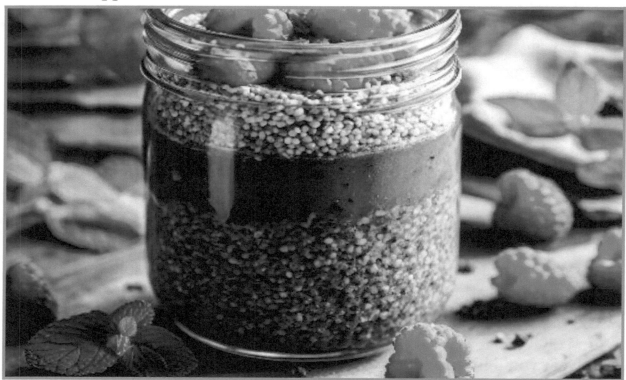

Instructions:

1. Mix the Ingredients: In a medium bowl, whisk together the almond milk, chia seeds, cocoa powder, maple syrup or honey, and vanilla extract until well combined.
2. Refrigerate: Cover the bowl and refrigerate for at least 4 hours or overnight, allowing the chia seeds to absorb the liquid and create a pudding-like consistency. Stir once after the first 30 minutes to prevent clumping.
3. Serve: Divide the pudding into two serving bowls or glasses.
4. Add Toppings (Optional): Top with fresh berries, a sprinkle of shaved dark chocolate, or a dollop of whipped cream for added indulgence.
5. Enjoy: Serve chilled for a rich and creamy treat.

Nutrition Information (per serving):

- Calories: 140
- Protein: 4g
- Carbohydrates: 15g
- Fat: 7g
- Fiber: 5g
- Sugar: 7g

Points Value: 4 WW Points per serving

Tips & Variations:

- Sweeter Option: Add an extra teaspoon of sweetener if you prefer a sweeter pudding.
- Dairy-Free Topping: Use coconut whipped cream for a dairy-free garnish.
- Meal Prep: Make in advance and store in the fridge for up to 3 days for a quick grab-and-go dessert.

This Dark Chocolate Chia Pudding is proof that you can enjoy rich, chocolatey desserts while staying aligned with your health goals. With its creamy texture and bold flavor, it's a guilt-free indulgence you'll crave.

Apple Cinnamon Oatmeal

This Apple Cinnamon Oatmeal is warm, comforting, and packed with the flavors of sweet apples and spicy cinnamon. It's a perfect dessert or breakfast option that feels indulgent but is incredibly healthy.

- Prep Time: 5 minutes
- Cook Time: 10 minutes
- Total Time: 15 minutes
- Servings: 2

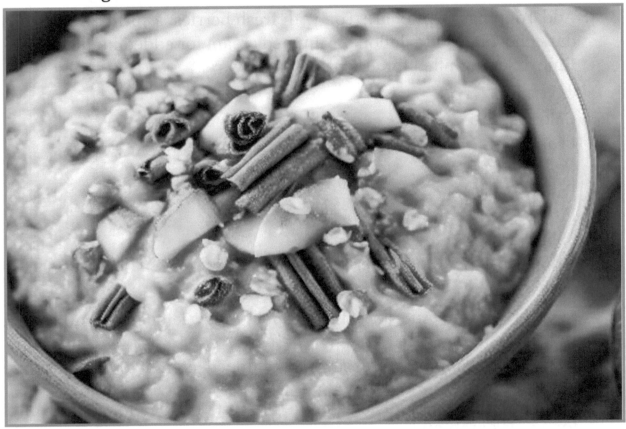

Ingredients:

- 1 cup old-fashioned rolled oats
- 2 cups unsweetened almond milk or water
- 1 medium apple, diced
- 1 tablespoon honey or maple syrup
- 1/2 teaspoon ground cinnamon
- 1/4 teaspoon ground nutmeg

- 1/4 teaspoon vanilla extract
- 1 tablespoon chopped walnuts or pecans (optional)
- Optional toppings: Additional diced apple, raisins, or a sprinkle of cinnamon

Instructions:

1. Cook the Oats: In a medium saucepan, combine the rolled oats and almond milk. Bring to a boil over medium heat, then reduce to a simmer.
2. Add the Apples and Spices: Stir in the diced apple, honey or maple syrup, cinnamon, nutmeg, and vanilla extract. Cook for 5-7 minutes, stirring occasionally, until the oats are creamy and the apples are tender.
3. Serve and Garnish: Divide the oatmeal into bowls and garnish with chopped walnuts or pecans and additional diced apple, if desired. Serve warm.

Nutrition Information (per serving):

- Calories: 180
- Protein: 5g
- Carbohydrates: 30g
- Fat: 4g
- Fiber: 5g
- Sugar: 12g

Points Value: 4 WW Points per serving

Tips & Variations:

- Dairy-Free Option: Use coconut milk or soy milk instead of almond milk.
- Extra Sweetness: Add a few raisins or a drizzle of maple syrup for added sweetness.
- Make Ahead: Prepare the oatmeal in advance and reheat for a quick dessert or breakfast.

This Apple Cinnamon Oatmeal is a warm, comforting dessert that feels like a hug in a bowl. With its natural sweetness and creamy texture, it's a guilt-free indulgence perfect for any time of the day.

Banana Nice Cream

This Banana Nice Cream is a creamy, dairy-free alternative to traditional ice cream. Made with just bananas and optional add-ins, it's a quick and healthy way to enjoy a frozen treat without added sugar or guilt.

- Prep Time: 5 minutes
- Freeze Time: 2 hours
- Total Time: 2 hours 5 minutes
- Servings: 2

Ingredients:

- 2 ripe bananas, sliced and frozen
- 1/2 teaspoon vanilla extract
- Optional add-ins: 1 tablespoon unsweetened cocoa powder, a handful of frozen berries, or a tablespoon of peanut butter
- Optional toppings: Chopped nuts, dark chocolate shavings, or fresh fruit

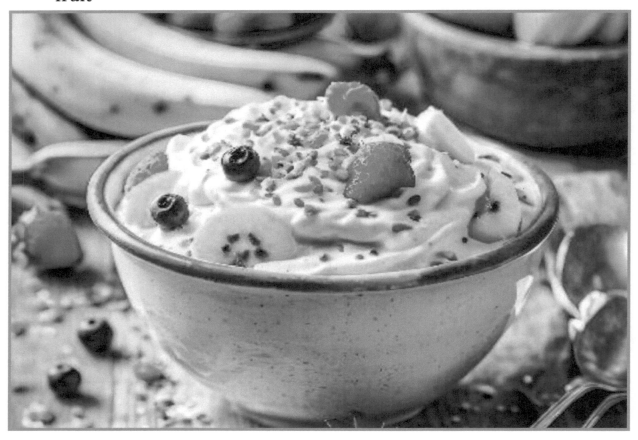

Instructions:

1. Prepare the Bananas: Peel and slice the ripe bananas, then freeze them in a single layer on a baking sheet for at least 2 hours or until completely frozen.
2. Blend the Nice Cream: Place the frozen banana slices in a food processor or high-speed blender. Blend until smooth and creamy, scraping down the sides as needed. Add the vanilla extract and any optional add-ins, blending until incorporated.
3. Serve and Enjoy: Scoop the nice cream into bowls and serve immediately. Garnish with your favorite toppings, if desired.

Nutrition Information (per serving):

- Calories: 120
- Protein: 1g
- Carbohydrates: 30g
- Fat: 0g
- Fiber: 3g
- Sugar: 19g

Points Value: 2 WW Points per serving

Tips & Variations:

- Extra Creaminess: Add a splash of almond milk while blending if the mixture is too thick.
- Chocolate Banana Nice Cream: Blend in 1 tablespoon of unsweetened cocoa powder for a chocolatey twist.
- Make Ahead: Store in the freezer for up to a week. Let it sit at room temperature for 5 minutes before scooping.

This Banana Nice Cream is a refreshing and creamy dessert that satisfies your sweet tooth with just a few simple ingredients. It's a versatile and healthy alternative to ice cream that you can enjoy anytime.

Chapter 8: Snacks & Smoothies

Snacks and smoothies are essential for maintaining energy and curbing hunger between meals. These recipes are designed to be nutritious, portable, and easy to prepare, making them ideal for busy days or on-the-go lifestyles.

Hummus Veggie Sticks

This Hummus Veggie Sticks recipe is a simple, nutritious snack that's as convenient as it is delicious. With crunchy vegetables and creamy hummus, it's a perfect balance of textures and flavors.

- Prep Time: 10 minutes
- Cook Time: 0 minutes
- Total Time: 10 minutes
- Servings: 4

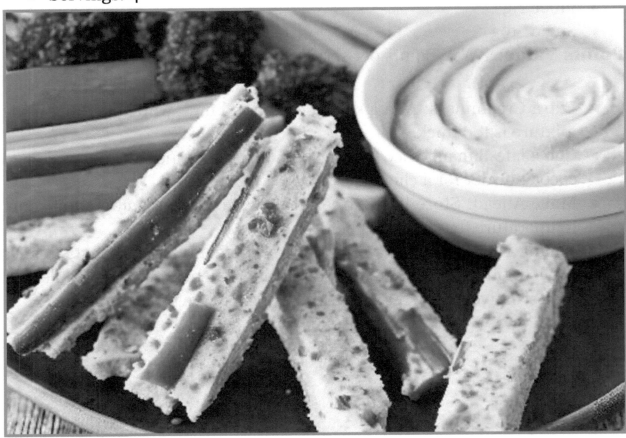

Ingredients:

- 1 cup hummus (store-bought or homemade)
- 1 cup carrot sticks
- 1 cup celery sticks
- 1 cup cucumber sticks
- 1 cup bell pepper strips (red, yellow, or green)

Instructions:

- Prepare the Vegetables: Wash and cut the vegetables into sticks or strips for easy dipping.
- Serve with Hummus: Arrange the vegetables on a platter or in individual snack containers. Serve with a portion of hummus for dipping.

Nutrition Information (per serving):

- Calories: 120
- Protein: 4g
- Carbohydrates: 12g
- Fat: 7g
- Fiber: 4g
- Sugar: 4g

Points Value: 3 WW Points per serving

Tips & Variations:

- Homemade Hummus: Blend 1 can of chickpeas, 2 tablespoons tahini, 1 clove garlic, 2 tablespoons lemon juice, and a pinch of salt for a quick homemade version.
- Add Crunch: Include other veggies like snap peas, radishes, or broccoli florets.
- Spice It Up: Sprinkle the hummus with smoked paprika or red pepper flakes for added flavor.

Hummus Veggie Sticks are a convenient and nutritious way to enjoy a crunchy, creamy snack. Perfect for prepping ahead, they make a great addition to your daily routine.

Nutty Trail Mix

This Nutty Trail Mix is a customizable, nutrient-packed snack that's perfect for curbing hunger on the go. Packed with healthy fats, fiber, and natural sweetness, it's a satisfying way to stay fueled between meals.

- Prep Time: 5 minutes
- Cook Time: 0 minutes
- Total Time: 5 minutes
- Servings: 4

Ingredients:

- 1/2 cup raw almonds
- 1/2 cup raw cashews
- 1/4 cup sunflower seeds
- 1/4 cup unsweetened dried cranberries
- 1/4 cup dark chocolate chips or cacao nibs
- 1/4 teaspoon cinnamon (optional)

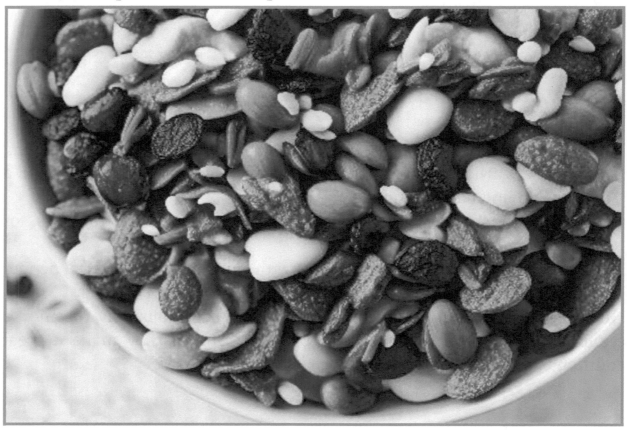

Instructions:

1. Combine Ingredients: In a large bowl, mix the almonds, cashews, sunflower seeds, dried cranberries, and dark chocolate chips. Add a sprinkle of cinnamon if desired.
2. Portion the Mix: Divide the trail mix into 4 individual portions for easy snacking.
3. Store: Store in airtight containers or snack bags for up to 2 weeks.

Nutrition Information (per serving):

- Calories: 200
- Protein: 5g
- Carbohydrates: 15g
- Fat: 13g
- Fiber: 3g
- Sugar: 6g

Points Value: 5 WW Points per serving

Tips & Variations:

- Nut-Free Option: Replace nuts with roasted chickpeas or pumpkin seeds for a nut-free version.
- Extra Sweetness: Add a few chopped dried apricots or dates for more natural sweetness.
- Customizable: Mix in your favorite nuts, seeds, or dried fruits to create your perfect blend.

Nutty Trail Mix is a versatile, nutrient-rich snack that's perfect for busy days, hiking trips, or simply enjoying at home. It's a great way to fuel your body with wholesome ingredients.

Green Detox Smoothie

This Green Detox Smoothie is a nutrient-packed blend of fresh fruits and greens that's as delicious as it is energizing. It's perfect for a morning boost or a refreshing snack any time of day.

- Prep Time: 5 minutes

- Cook Time: 0 minutes
- Total Time: 5 minutes
- Servings: 2

Ingredients:

- 1 cup fresh spinach or kale
- 1 small green apple, cored and chopped
- 1/2 cucumber, peeled and chopped
- 1/2 banana, frozen
- 1/2 cup unsweetened almond milk or coconut water
- 1/2 cup water or ice
- 1 tablespoon lemon juice
- 1/2 teaspoon grated fresh ginger (optional)

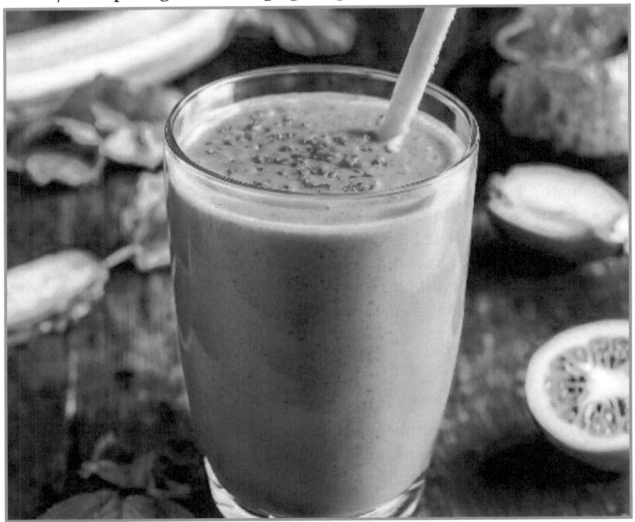

Instructions:

- Blend the Ingredients: In a blender, combine the spinach or kale, green apple, cucumber, banana, almond milk or coconut water, water or ice, lemon juice, and ginger if using. Blend until smooth.
- Serve Immediately: Pour the smoothie into two glasses and serve immediately for the freshest flavor and texture.

Nutrition Information (per serving):

- Calories: 90
- Protein: 2g
- Carbohydrates: 20g
- Fat: 0.5g
- Fiber: 4g
- Sugar: 10g

Points Value: 2 WW Points per serving

Tips & Variations:

- Sweeter Option: Add a teaspoon of honey or a couple of pitted dates if you prefer a sweeter smoothie.
- Extra Protein: Add a scoop of protein powder for a more filling snack.
- Dairy-Free Alternative: Use oat milk or rice milk instead of almond milk.

This Green Detox Smoothie is a light, refreshing, and nutrient-dense option that's perfect for starting your day or recharging in the afternoon. Its vibrant flavor and creamy texture make it a go-to healthy drink.

Oat Peanut Energy Bites

These Oat Peanut Energy Bites are a no-bake, portable snack that's packed with protein, fiber, and natural sweetness. Perfect for meal prep, they'll keep you fueled and satisfied on busy days.

- Prep Time: 10 minutes
- Chill Time: 30 minutes
- Total Time: 40 minutes
- Servings: 12 bites

Ingredients:

- 1 cup old-fashioned rolled oats
- 1/2 cup natural peanut butter
- 1/4 cup honey or maple syrup
- 1/4 cup ground flaxseed or chia seeds
- 1/4 cup mini dark chocolate chips
- 1/2 teaspoon vanilla extract
- Pinch of salt

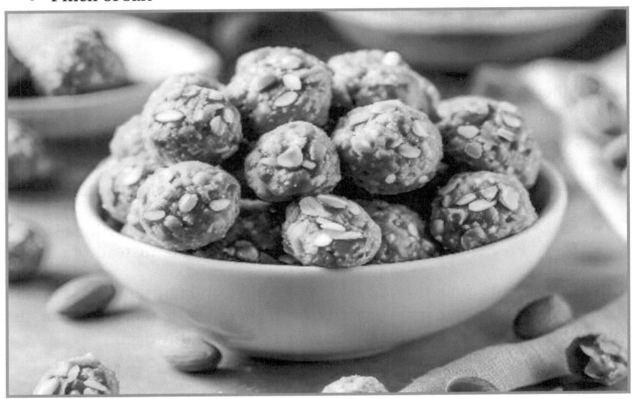

Instructions:

- Mix the Ingredients: In a large bowl, combine the rolled oats, peanut butter, honey or maple syrup, ground flaxseed or chia seeds, chocolate chips, vanilla extract, and salt. Stir until well combined.
- Chill the Mixture: Cover the bowl and refrigerate for 30 minutes to make the mixture easier to handle.
- Form the Bites: Roll the mixture into 12 evenly sized balls using your hands. Place them on a baking sheet or plate lined with parchment paper.

- Serve or Store: Enjoy immediately, or store the bites in an airtight container in the fridge for up to one week.

Nutrition Information (per bite):

- Calories: 120
- Protein: 3g
- Carbohydrates: 12g
- Fat: 6g
- Fiber: 2g
- Sugar: 6g

Points Value: 3 WW Points per bite

Tips & Variations:

- Nut-Free Option: Use sunflower seed butter instead of peanut butter for a nut-free version.
- Flavor Boost: Add a sprinkle of cinnamon or a dash of cocoa powder for extra flavor.
- Make Ahead: These bites freeze well; store them in the freezer for up to 2 months and thaw before eating.

Oat Peanut Energy Bites are a convenient and delicious way to stay fueled throughout the day. With their perfect balance of sweetness and texture, they're a snack you'll love to have on hand.

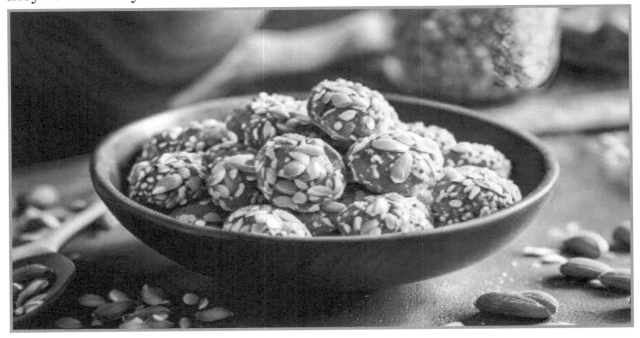

Conclusion

Congratulations on taking the first step toward a healthier and more balanced lifestyle! This cookbook was designed with you in mind—packed with flavorful, satisfying recipes that align with your goals and make the process of eating well enjoyable and sustainable.

—From hearty breakfasts to indulgent desserts, you've explored a variety of dishes that show how nourishing your body doesn't have to mean sacrificing flavor or enjoyment. Whether you're savoring a comforting soup, whipping up a vibrant salad, or indulging in a guilt-free dessert, every recipe in this collection was crafted to inspire confidence in the kitchen and delight at the table.

A Few Parting Tips:

- Meal Prep for Success: Plan ahead to ensure you always have healthy, delicious options on hand. Many of the recipes in this cookbook are perfect for meal prepping, so you're never caught off guard.
- Balance and Flexibility: Remember, no single meal or food choice defines your journey. Embrace balance and enjoy the process of discovering what works best for you.
- Experiment and Customize: Use these recipes as a foundation to get creative. Swap ingredients, add your own twists, and make these dishes truly your own.
- Celebrate Progress: Every small step counts. Celebrate your victories—whether it's mastering a new recipe or reaching a personal milestone.

A Lifelong Love for Healthy Eating

Healthy eating isn't about restrictions; it's about creating a lifestyle filled with foods that nourish your body and bring you joy. With the recipes and ideas in this cookbook, you have the tools to make every meal a celebration of wellness.

—Thank you for letting this cookbook be part of your journey. Here's to flavorful meals, exciting discoveries, and a future filled with health and happiness. Bon appétit!

Made in United States
Troutdale, OR
01/30/2025